Ultrasound
Differential Diagnosis

Ultrasound Differential Diagnosis

Satish K Bhargava
MBBS MD (Radiodiagnosis) MD (Radiotherapy)
DMRD FICRI FIAMS FCCP FUSI FIMSA FAMS
Professor and Head
Department of Radiology and Imaging
University College of Medical Sciences
(University of Delhi) and GTB Hospital
Delhi

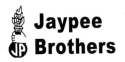
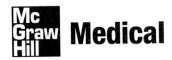

© 2007 Satish K Bhargava

First published in India by

Jaypee Brothers Medical Publishers (P) Ltd
EMCA House, 23/23B Ansari Road, Daryaganj
New Delhi 110 002, India
Phones: +91-11-23272143, +91-11-23272703, +91-11-23282021, +91-11-23245672
Fax: +91-11-23276490, +91-11-23245683   e-mail: jaypee@jaypeebrothers.com
Visit our website: www.jaypeebrothers.com

First published in USA by The McGraw-Hill Companies, 2 Penn Plaza, New York, NY 10121-2298.
Exclusively worldwide distributor except South Asia (India, Nepal, Sri Lanka, Bhutan, Pakistan,
Bangladesh).

NOTICE

Medicine is an ever-changing science. As new research and clinical experience broaden our knowledge, changes in treatment and drug therapy are required. The authors and the publisher of this work
have checked with sources believed to be reliable in their efforts to provide information that is complete
and generally in accord with the standards accepted at the time of publication. However, in view of the
possibility of human error changes in medical science, neither the editors nor the publisher nor any
other party who has been involved in the preparation or publication of this work warrants that the
information contained herein is in every respect accurate or complete, and they disclaim all respon-
sibility for any errors or omissions or for the results obtained from use of the information contained in
this work. Readers are encouraged to confirm the information contained herein with other sources. For
example and in particular, readers are advised to check the product information sheet included in the
package of each drug they plan to administer to be certain that the information contained in this work
is accurate and that changes have not been made in the recommended dose or in the contraindications
for administration. This recommendation is of particular importance in connection with new or infrequently used drugs.

ISBN   0-07-148575-9
ISBN 13   9780071485753

*Dedicated to
My loving late wife
Kalpana
and my son
Sumeet
Whose inspiration and sacrifice
have made possible to
bring out this book*

Contributors

Satish K Bhargava
Professor and Head
Department of Radiology and Imaging
University College of Medical Sciences
(University of Delhi) and GTB Hospital
Delhi

Sumeet Bhargava
LLR Medical College
Meerut (UP)

Shuchi Bhatt
Sr Lecturer
Department of Radiology and Imaging
University College of Medical Sciences
(University of Delhi) and GTB Hospital
Delhi

Parul Garg
Sr Resident
Department of Radiology and Imaging
University College of Medical Sciences
(University of Delhi) and GTB Hospital
Delhi

Pushpender Gupta
Resident
Department of Radiology and Imaging
University College of Medical Sciences
(University of Delhi) and GTB Hospital
Delhi

Puneet Singh Kochar
Resident
Department of Radiology and Imaging
University College of Medical Sciences
(University of Delhi) and GTB Hospital
Delhi

Pardeep Kumar
Resident
Department of Radiology and Imaging
University College of Medical Sciences
(University of Delhi) and GTB Hospital
Delhi

Sapna Maheshwari (Somani)
Sr Resident
Department of Radiology and Imaging
University College of Medical Sciences
(University of Delhi) and GTB Hospital
Delhi

Gopesh Mehrotra
Reader
Department of Radiology and Imaging
University College of Medical Sciences
(University of Delhi) and GTB Hospital
Delhi

Mamta Motla
Sr Resident
Department of Radiology and Imaging
University College of Medical Sciences
(University of Delhi) and GTB Hospital
Delhi

Rajul Rastogi
Sr Resident
Department of Radiology and Imaging
University College of Medical Sciences
(University of Delhi) and GTB Hospital
Delhi

Ruchi Rastogi
Sr Resident
Department of Cardiac Radiology
All India Institute of Medical Sciences
Ansari Nagar, New Delhi

Vinita Rathi
Associate Professor
Department of Radiology and Imaging
University College of Medical Sciences
(University of Delhi) and GTB Hospital
Delhi

Anubhav Sarikwal
Sr Resident
Department of Radiodiagnosis and Imaging
University College of Medical Sciences
(University of Delhi) and GTB Hospital
Delhi

Ashish Verma
Sr Resident
Department of Radiodiagnosis and Imaging
Sanjay Gandhi Postgraduate Institute of Medical
Sciences
Rai Bareli Road
Lucknow (UP)

Preface

Since the introduction of US, this modality has evolved from its primitive nature to its present glamorous status. Its popularity in radiology has always been due to its cost effectiveness, easy availability and noninvasive nature. Its diagnostic role has been explored in every organ system and its usefulness felt every time. Its support in therapeutic techniques is unparalleled. Radiology without ultrasound is unimaginable.

Almost always realtime US is the initial investigative tool in the radiology department. Many a time this modality is enough to establish a diagnosis and always provides a direction for further evaluation. Its uniqueness lies in its operator-dependent nature. As the ultrasonologist scans through the region of interest recognition and interpretation of the important findings are important for establishing and imaging diagnosis. It is also imperative to know the various conditions producing a particular sonographic finding. The only ultraound can be judiciously used to answer the question posed to the radiologist. This book is a special effort to provide a concise knowledge of the differential diagnosis of a sonographic finding. A list of the various clinical conditions and their short description is the main feature of the text. The information has been kept concise and unnecessary repetition avoided. Line diagrams and illustrations have been added to support the text. The aim of this book is to assist the sonologist with logical interpretation of the scan. I hope this attempt will prove useful to all practising sonologists.

Satish K Bhargava

Acknowledgements

I am grateful to my colleagues and friends who gave timely support and stood solidly behind me in our joint endeavour of bringing out this book which was required keeping in view of wide acceptability of ultrasound in developing countries like ours. My special heartfelt thanks are due to the sincere and hardworking staff of M/s Jaypee Brothers Medical Publishers (P) Ltd., New Delhi particularly Shri Jitendar P Vij, Chairman and Managing Director, Mr Tarun Duneja, General Manager Publishing, Mr PS Ghuman, Senior Production Manager, Mrs Yashu Kapoor, DTP Operator and Ms Mubeen Bano. It is indeed the result of the hard work of the staff of M/s Jaypee Brothers and the contributors who have always been in keen desire to work with smiling faces and with polite voices as a result of which this book has seen the light of day.

Contents

1

Chest

Ultrasound is a noninvasive, relatively inexpensive and most rewarding imaging modality, carries no radiation burden, but not much exploited for evaluation of chest disease because of basic (inherent) properties of US waves not to pass through bony cage and air filled lungs. However, over a couple of years, US has emerged as a useful tool in evaluating wide range of perplexing clinical problems of chest due to presence of fluid in pleural space, consolidating or atelectatic lung or even tumor, provide window for US to penetrate and this has helped in diagnosis of certain conditions or limit the DD of conditions under consideration.

1. *Chest wall:* It has helped in diagnosing soft tissue abscesses, masses, osteomyelitis, rib tumors and even fracture where plain X-ray gives only soft tissue swelling or obliteration of costophrenic angle (may be due to pleural fluid or sometimes by rib tumor) and also where rib erosion is due to underlying carcinoma. Sometimes, when clinically mass is suspected with fractures, US can be used as

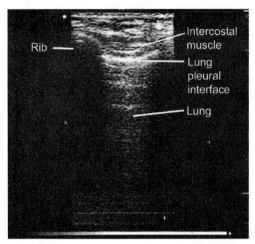

Fig. 1.1.1: Normal lung as seen in transverse section. Ribs with distal shadowing are shown with intercostal muscles. The lung pleural interface is seen as an echogenic line

a first modality particularly in children to avoid radiation by getting an X-ray chest

2. *Mediastinum:* Anterior mediastinum can be very well evaluated by US through suprasternal route by elevating shoulders and extending the neck. This will avoid radiation particularly in children where it is due to thymus. Even paratracheal and hilar adenopathy can be diagnosed especially in tubercular patients where it is not only helpful in diagnosis but also in follow-up when child is on anti-tubercular therapy, thus avoiding unnecessary radiation and getting repeated X-rays.

3. *Lung parenchyma:* It is also helpful in differentiating consolidation, collapse and tumor of lung. A tumor

on US gives heterogeneous shadows, consolidation gives fluid bronchogram and collapse will give homogeneous shadow. Also it is helpful in differentiating solid vs cystic that is whether it is a hydatid cyst/thoracic kidney, etc. or a lung consolidation. Also it is helpful when X-ray chest PA view shows a homogeneous shadow in right lower zone—may be due to consolidation/hiatus hernia.

i. It is also a good screening modality in opaque hemithorax—due to collapse, large consolidation, tumor of lung or even tumour from bony cage because of different US spectrum.

ii. It is also a good modality for diagnosing diaphragmatic pathologies and lesions above

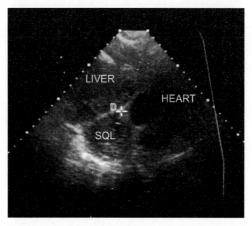

Fig. 1.1.2: Lung sequestration—predominantly hypoechoic SOL with air bronchogram in it is seen in right lower lobe of lung adjacent to the heart in this case of nonresolving pneumonia in 16 years old patient

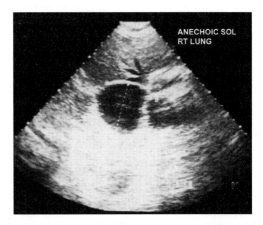

Fig. 1.1.3: Lung hydatid seen as anechoic cystic
lesion in transverse scan of lung

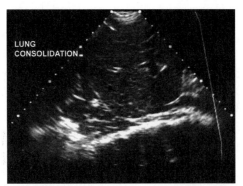

Fig. 1.1.4: Consolidation—seen as a homogeneous hypoechoic lesion with air bronchogram in right lower lobe of lung

(pleural fluid/consolidation) or below (subpulmonic effusion).

4. *Pleura:* US is a good modality to differentiate pleural
lesions from parenchymal ones. It is also helpful in

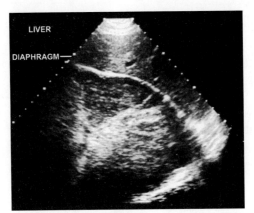

Fig. 1.1.5: Lung abscess—a large predominantly hypoechoic SOL with internal septae and posterior enhancement is seen in lower lobe of right lung. Aspiration revealed pus. Inversion of diaphragm is seen

diagnosing minimal amount of fluid in pleural cavity, even 5-10 ml of fluid, thus avoiding need of lateral decubitus film/lateral chest film.

i. It also gives the etiology of pleural fluid due to its appearance as anechoic, hypoechoic, echogenic, presence of debris, nodules and types of septa.

ii. Anechoic—all transudates are anechoic, however all anechoic collections are not transudates. About one-third of exudative collection tends to be anechoic in the beginning.

iii. Hypoechoic—usually exudative effusions, empyema and later stages of hemothorax.

iv. Echogenic—hemothorax or empyema.

v. Debris—represents settled down pus cell, blood cells, etc.

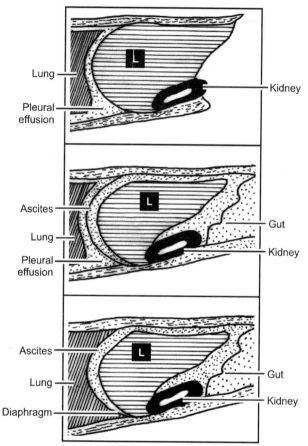

Fig. 1.1.6: A. Pleural effusion superior to the diaphragm B. Pleural effusion and ascites outlining the diaphragm. C. Ascites only. Irregular outline of the gut is seen due to ascites

    vi. Septations—usually represent process of locu-
lation and fibrosis occurring in pleural effusion.
Thin clean septa with no or very minimal

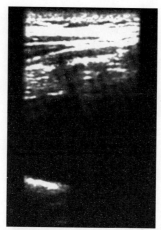

Fig. 1.1.7: Longitudinal intercostal view in a patient with pleural effusion showing echogenic surface of visceral and perietal pleura

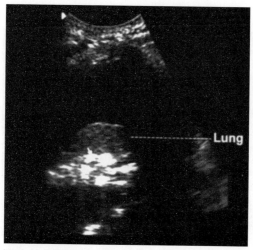

Fig. 1.1.8: Longitudinal intercostal view—pleural effusion and collapsed lung showing echogenic gas filled bronchus (arrow) within the collapsed lung

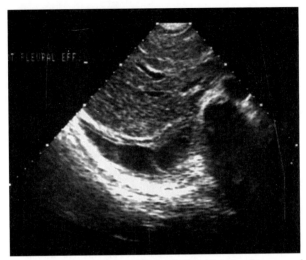

Fig. 1.1.9: Loculated multiseptated fluid collection seen in the pleural cavity with associated pleural thickening

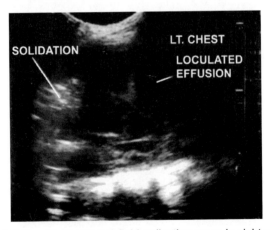

Fig. 1.1.10: Multiseptated fluid collection seen in right pleural cavity in the case of infected pleural effusion

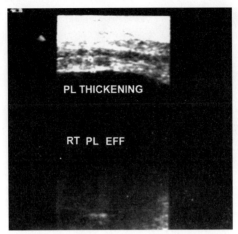

PL THICKENING

RT PL EFF

Fig. 1.1.11: Thickened pleura seen along with pleural effusion

       debris— tubercular pleural effusion. However, thick, shaggy irregular septations with debris— pyogenic effusion.

vii. Pleural nodule/masses—represent mesothelioma, metastatic nodule and tuberculomata. In addition to characteristics septations the thickness of parietal pleura and combined (parietal + visceral) also give etiological diagnosis. As tubercular pleural effusion—parietal pleural thickness varies 2-8 mm and combined pleural varies from 4-10 mm. In pyogenic pleural effusion—parietal pleural thickness varies from 5-22 mm and combined 8-27 mm. In hemothoraces (post-traumatic) thick irregular mantle of pleura around hypoechoic pleural collection is seen, pleural thickness varies from 12-18 mm.

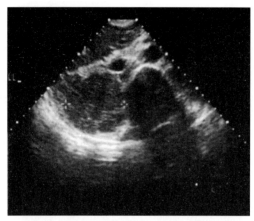

Fig. 1.1.12: A predominantly hypoechoic solid mass lesion seen in right lower lobe of lung

5. *Intervention*—US is very helpful in fine needle aspiration biopsy, pleural tapping, guided pleural aspiration and tube placement.
6. *ICU*—US is very helpful in critically ill-patients that is trauma and ICU—needs serial X-rays to see day to day changes in lesions—particularly when there is inability to position the patient as required and usually substandard quality of X-rays.

Limitations

- Pneumothoraces/hydropneumothorax
- Limited information about mediastinum, hilar and proximal airways
- Restricted field of view
- Familiarity of clinician
- Operator dependent

Other Advantages

- Lower cost
- Increase flexibility
- No radiation
- Good guidance tool
- Repeated evaluation with no radiation cost.

Ability to detect abdominal lesions associated with causative of chest lesion as liver abscesses leading to pleural effusion.

1.2 PLEURAL EFFUSION

Pleural effusion can be transudative or exudative.

Signs of pleural fluid on USG—transudative effusion—

Pleural (fluid) that changes shape with respiration.

Exudative effusion—

Fluid with floating echodensities

Septations—thick and shaggy

Fibrin strands

May be anechoic fluid

Echogenic fluid

Pleural nodules

Thickened pleura

Causes of Transudative Pleural Effusion

1. Increased hydrostatic pressure
   - Congestive heart failure
   - SVC obstruction
   - Constrictive pericarditis

2. Decreased osmotic pressure
   - Cirrhosis with ascites
   - Peritoneal dialysis
   - Acute glomerulonephritis
   - Nephrotic syndrome
   - Urinary tract obstruction
   - Hypoalbuminemia
   - Overhydration
   - Hypothyroidism

Causes of Exudative Pleural Effusion

1. Infection
   - Parapneumonic effusion
   - Empyema
   - Tuberculosis
   - Fungi (*Nocardia,* actinomycosis)
2. Neoplasm
   - Pleural metastasis
   - Pleural mesothelioma
   - Bronchogenic carcinoma
   - Lymphoma
3. Vascular
   - Pulmonary emboli
4. Collagen Vascular Disease
   - SLE
   - Rheumatoid arthritis
5. Abdominal Disease
   - Subphrenic abscess
   - Pancreatitis

6. Trauma
   • Hydrothorax
7. Miscellaneous
   • Drug induced effusion

1.3 PLEURAL PLAQUE

Common causes of pleural plaque includes:
• Pneumonia
• Asbestos exposure
• Pulmonary infarction
• Trauma
• Chemical pleurodesis
• Drug related pleural disease

Plaques resulting from asbestos exposure are usually confined to the parietal pleura. Ultrasound demonstrates pleural plaques as smooth, elliptical, hypoechoic pleural thickening.

Visceral pleural plaques are differentiated from parietal pleura by observing the 'gliding sign' during respiration.

Calcified pleural plaques are irregular, echogenic and produce acoustic shadowing and comet tail artifact.

1.4 PLEURAL MASSES

1. Loculated pleural effusion
2. Metastasis
3. Malignant mesothelioma
4. Pleural fibroma
5. Fibrin balls

Loculated Pleural Effusion

Anechoic collection seen within the pleural cavity.

Metastasis

Pleural effusion associated with malignant disease may result from:

Malignant cell implantation on the pleura (common causes: lung, breast and GIT cancers).

Obstruction of pleura or pulmonary lymphatics (common causes: lymphoma, breast cancer).

Obstruction of pulmonary veins usually by lung cancers.

Malignant cells shed freely into pleural space

Obstruction of thoracic ducts, resulting in chylous effusion. (usually due to lymphoma)

Sonographic findings favoring malignant etiology.

- Solid nodules in the pleural space
- Circumferential pleural thickening
- Nodular pleural thickening or >1 cm pleural thickening.
- Pleural thickening involving the mediastinal pleura.

Pleural Mesothelioma

Malignant mesothelioma is a rare and usually fatal pleural tumors associated with asbestos exposure.

Imaging Findings

Diffuse pleural thickening, often nodular and irregular (86%)

Calcification in pleura (74%)
Focal pleural mass (25%)
Rib destruction occurs with advanced disease.

Pleural Fibroma (Local Benign Mesothelioma)

A smooth lobular mass, 2-15 cm diameter arising more frequently from the visceral pleura.

Pedunculated mass changes shape with respiration (30-50%).

Forms an obtuse angle with the chest wall.

Fibrin Balls

These develop in serofibrinous pleural effusion and become visible following absorption of fluid.

Small and tend to be situated near the lung base.

• May disappear spontaneously or remain unchanged for many years.

1.5 MEDIASTINAL LYMPHADENOPATHY

Tuberculosis	Sarcoidosis	Lymphoma
Unilateral	Bilateral	Bilateral
—	Symmetric	Asymmetric
Right paratracheal and tracheobronchial nodes are most commonly involved	— Bilateral hilar with or without right paratracheal, aortopulmonary window lymphadenopathy.	Superior mediastinum most common site with or without unilateral or bilateral hilar nodes

Contd...

Contd...

	— Mediastinal LN with or without hilar LN—unusual. — Characteristic involvement of bronchopulmonary nodes.	— in NHL involvement of other nodal groups (cardiophrenic, posterior mediastinal) also seen more commonly than HD
Low attenuation	Isodense	Isodense
Mild homogeneous enhancement to rim enhancement	Homogeneous mild to moderate enhancement	Mild homogeneous enhancement
May show calcification	May show rim calcification	Calcification unusual without treatment
More likely to be confluent	Discrete	Usually discrete May be confluent with large nodal masses

1.6 VASCULAR LESIONS OF MEDIASTINUM

Ultrasound is an excellent, noninvasive method of diagnosing masses of vascular origin in the mediastinum.

Vascular nature of a suspected mass can be confirmed by ultrasound using imaging supplemented by color flow and spectral Doppler effect—

• Tortuous brachiocephalic artery
• Aneurysm of the aorta

- Aneurysm of the sinus of Valsalva
- Right sided aortic arch
- Double aortic arch
- Dilated superior vena cava.

1.7 CYSTIC MASSES OF MEDIASTINUM

1. Congenital cyst (Benign)
   - Bronchogenic cyst
   - Pericardial cyst
   - Esophageal duplication cyst
   - Neuroenteric cyst
   - Thymic cyst
2. Mature cystic teratoma
3. Meningocele (Lateral)
4. Lymphangioma
5. Cystic degeneration
   - Hodgkin's disease
   - Metastasis to lymph nodes
   - Nerve root tumors
6. Mediastinal abscess
7. Pancreatic pseudocyst

Ultrasonography can be useful in evaluating a mass adjacent to pleural surface or cardiophrenic angle. At US, the benign cysts typically appear as anechoic thin walled masses with increased through transmission.

- Ultrasound is used to characterize wall thickness, septations, vascularity, appearance of internal fluid, location and relationship to adjacent structures.

Pericardial cyst—results from aberrations in the formation of celomic cavities. Pericardial cysts are invariably connected to the pericardium but only a few cases unable to show communication with the pericardial sac.

The majority of pericardial cysts arise in anterior cardiophrenic, more commonly on the right side. Occasionally cysts are pedunculated.

Mature Cystic Teratoma

These are cystic tumors composed of well differentiated derivations from at least two of the three germ layers. Majority of dermoid cysts are in the anterior mediastinum.

Most cystic teratoma are multilocular but unilocular cystic lesions also occur.

They may contain four types of tissues-including fluid, fat, soft tissues, calcium but fluid containing cystic component are usually prominent.

A fat fluid level within the mass is highly specific finding but is seen less frequently.

Cystic Degeneration

Many tumors and lymph nodes can undergo cystic degeneration and demonstrate mixed solid and cystic elements. If degeneration is extensive, the appearance of the lesion is indistinguishable from those of a congenital cyst. Cystic degeneration of a solid mass is more likely to occur after radiation therapy or chemotherapy but may be seen prior to treatment.

- A mediastinal abscess or pancreatic pseudocyst appears as a fluid containing mediastinal cystic mass, but clinical features usually permit differentiation from true cysts or neoplasms.

1.8 DIAPHRAGM

Bilateral Diaphragmatic Elevation

a. Shallow inspiration (most common).

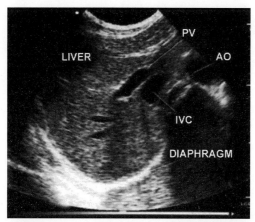

Fig. 1.8.1: Liver in transverse scan—right lobe of liver

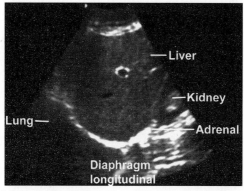

Fig. 1.8.2: Longitudinal image showing the various relation along the anteroposterior extent of the diaphragm on right side

b. Abdominal cause (USG useful by showing fluid, fetus or an abdominal mass as the cause)
   1. Obesity
   2. Pregnancy
   3. Ascites
   4. Any large abdominal mass.
c. Pulmonary causes-USG little use
   • Chext X-ray/CT required making the diagnosis.
d. Neuromuscular disorders
   1. Myasthenia gravis—chest CT may show thymoma.
   2. Amyotropic lateral sclerosis—USG is of little use.
      • MRI required for diagnosis.

Unilateral Diaphragmatic Elevation

Subpulmonic Pleural Effusion

• Ultrasound confirmatory
• Shows the presence of fluid is pleural cavity with normal relative position of bothdomes of diaphragm.

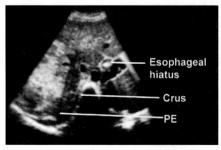

Fig. 1.8.3: Showing diaphragmatic hiatus for IVC, esophagus and aorta

Pulmonary Causes

- USG may show the presence of elevation of one dome of diaphragm as compared to other dome. However underlying lung is usually not evaluated by ultrasound.
- Chest X-ray/CT will confirm the cause for diaphragmatic elevation.

Phrenic Nerve Paralysis (Diaphragmatic Paralysis)

- May occur due to
  a. Primary lung tumor
  b. Malignant mediastinal
  c. Iatrogenic
  d. Idiopathic
- Diagnosis is made on USG by observing the absent or paradoxical movement on the affected side with usual or exaggerated excursion on the opposite side. Paradoxical movement can be elicited by the coughing or sniffing tests.

Abdominal Causes

- Subphrenic abscesses.
  - In appropriate clinical setting usually H/o surgery
  - USG shows—elevated hemidiaphragm
  - Reduced or absent movement of the ipsilateral diaphragm
  - Subdiaphragmatic anechoic or hypoechoic collection
  - Usually ipsilateral pleural effusion present.

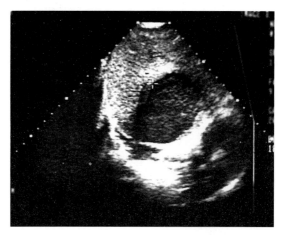

Fig. 1.8.4: Amebic liver abscess—a hypoechoic SOL is seen in the posterosuperior aspect of liver with evidence of posterior enhancement. It is extending into subdiaphragmatic space

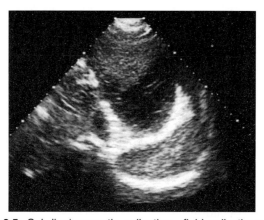

Fig. 1.8.5: Subdiaphragmatic collection—fluid collections with multiple internal septae is seen below the diaphragm

- Liver mass: (tumor, echinococcal cyst, abscess)
- Distended stomach or colon.
  Interposition of colon.

Diaphragmatic Hernia

- USG may show the discontinuity of the dome of diaphragm
- Bowel, spleen, kidney may be visualized inside thorax above dome of diaphragm
- Contralateral displacement of heart is visualised
- In congenital diaphragmatic hernia, polyhydramnios may be associated after 25 weeks.

Eventration of Diaphragm

- Complete—more commonly on left
- Partial—more commonly on right
- Complete eventration of diaphragm can be diagnosed by ultrasound
- Ultrasound in focal eventration shows evidence of typical focal diaphragmatic bulge filled by liver.

Diaphragmatic Rupture

- Traumatic—blunt or penetrating trauma
- Infection—ruptured amoebic liver abscess
- In post-traumatic rupture in large, usually over 10 cm, defects ultrasound may detect–disruption of diaphragmatic echoes. Herniation of abdominal viscera into thorax—associated pleural effusion. Sometimes—small diaphragmatic rents may be difficult to detect, but due to availability of high

frequency transducers, it is now possible to detect small disruption of diaphragmatic contour.

Neoplasms

- Very rarely diaphragmatic neoplasms
- Primary—various types of sarcomas
- Fibroma
- Secondary—Local invasion by adjacent pleural, peritoneal, thoracic and abdominal wall malignancies
- Distant metastasis from bronchogenic or ovarian cercinoma
- Wilms' tumor and osteogenic sarcoma are less common.

DIAPHRAGMATIC INVERSION

Normally diaphragm is convex towards thorax, but reverse occurs in inversion with convexity towards abdomen.

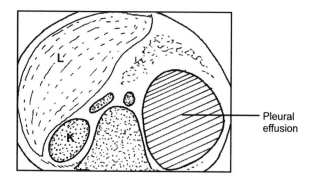

Fig. 1.8.6: Transverse view—a large pleural effusion inverting the diaphragm can look like a large cyst

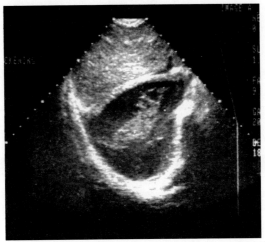

Fig. 1.8.7: Free fluid seen in right pleural cavity with collapsed lung inside—note the inverted diaphragm

- More common on left side, due to protective effect of liver on right side
- Part of diaphragm or entire diaphragm may be affected
- May occur due to large pleural effusion or neoplasm, pushing the diaphragm downwards
- May show little or asynchronous motion with respiration.

2

Neck Lesions

2.1 THYROID

2.1.1 SOLITARY THYROID NODULE

- Hyperplastic adenomatous nodule
- Adenoma
- Lymphoma
- Carcinoma

- USG features of benign goitrous nodules:
  - A thoroughly cystic appearance
  - Moving comet tail artefacts
  - Fluid-fluid level
  - Widespread cystic changes in iso-echoic or highly reflective nodules
  - Highly reflective nodules
  - A perilesional thin, uniform thickness echo-poor halo
  - Well defined and regular margins
  - Peripheral egg shell like or large coarse calcification
  - A perilesional blood flow pattern (Basket pattern)

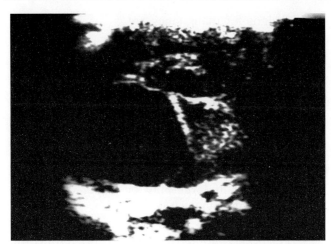

Fig. 2.1.1.1: A solitary thyroid nodule with homogenous paren-chyma in a euthyroid patient. Hypoechoic halo is visible around space occupying lesions

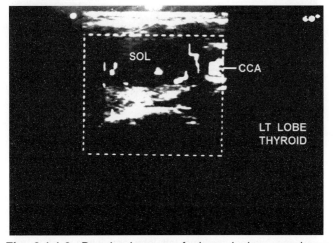

Fig. 2.1.1.2: Doppler images of above lesion reveals no vascularity in the mass but color flow corresponding to the halo is seen

- USG signs for malignancy are:
  - Low reflectivity
  - Irregular margins
  - Thick irregular halo
  - Microcalcification
  - Intranodal blood flow pattern
  - Hypervascularity
  - Vessel encasement
  - Invasion of vessels and adjacent structures
1. Hyperplastic or adenomatous nodule:
   - Isoechoic, if large-may be hyperechoic. Less commonly hypoechoic
   - Thin peripheral hyperechoic halo, complete
   - Perinodal blood flow. However, hyperfunctioning (Basket pattern)

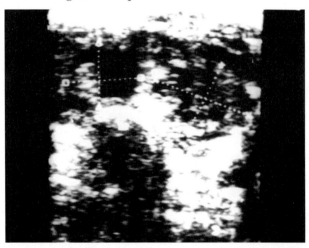

Fig. 2.1.1.3: Transverse scan neck showing multiple space occupying lesions involving left lobe and isthmus of thyroid. Cystic areas seen in nodules without calcification—multinodular goiter

- Adenomatous nodules frequently show both perinodal and intranodal vascularity
- May show degenerative changes:
  a. Purely an echoic—due to serous or colloid fluid.
  b. If hemorrhage occurs—echogenic fluid or fluid-fluid level may be present.
  c. If dense colloid material is present—comet tail artefect may be seen.
  d. Thin intracystic septation—which are avascular on Doppler study.
- Peripheral (egg shell like) or large and coarse calcification may be seen.

2. Adenomas:
- Solid, may be hyper, iso or hypoechoic
- Thick and smooth peripheral hypoechoic halo
- Spoke—and wheel like arrangement of vessels on Doppler study.

3. Lymphoma:
- Large hypoechoic lobulated mass which is nearly avascular
- May show large cystic areas due to necrosis
- May show encasement of neck vessels
- Heterogenous echotexture of remaining thyroid parenchyma due to associated chronic thyroiditis.

2.1.2 CARCINOMAS

Papillary Carcinoma

- 90 percent hypoechoic

- Microcalcifications may be present
- Hypervascularity, both intranodal and perinodal with disorganised arrangement of vessels on Doppler study
- Enlarged cervical lymph nodes due to metastasis, which may also show microcalcifications. Occasionally on USG cervical lymph node metastasis may be cystic.

Follicular Carcinoma

- Features similar to adenoma, except for
  - Irregular tumor margins
  - Thick irregular hypoechoic halo
  - Both intra- and perinodal vascularity with tortuous and choatic arrangement of internal blood vessels on color doppler.

Anaplastic Carcinoma Thyroid

- Large, hypoechoic
- Ill defined margins
- Encase or invade blood vessels and muscles in the neck.

Medullary Carcinoma Thyroid

- Sonographic appearance similar to papillary carcinoma (hypoechoic, irregular margins, hypervascularity) except that the local invasion and metastasis to cervical nodes occurs more frequently in patients with medullary carcinoma
- May show microcalcifications similar to papillary carcinoma

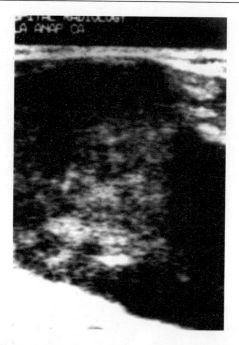

Fig. 2.1.2.1: Anaplastic carcinoma thyroid. Ultrasound image showing a large heteroechoic lesion involving right lobe of thyroid with brightly echogenic focus suggestive of calcification

- Familial in 20 percent patient and essential component of MEN type II syndrome.

2.1.3 THYROID CALCIFICATION

- Peripheral or egg shell like calcification is a feature of benign thyroid nodule
- Scattered large and coarse calcification is, if seen the nodule is more, likely to be benign

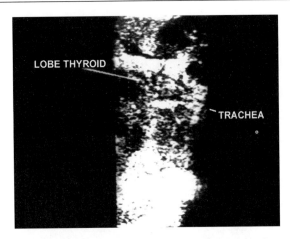

Fig. 2.1.2.2: Heterogenous multinodular parenchymal pattern of thyroid along with obscuration of anatomical planes seen in elderly patient. Discrete lymph nodes were also seen in post triangle

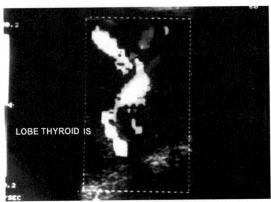

Fig. 2.1.2.3: Color velocity imaging revealed high velocity flow throughout the parenchyma suggestive of malignancy—medullary carcinoma

- Scattered fine and punctate calcifications (Micro-calcification) are seen in papillary carcinoma of thyroid (pemmoma bodies) or medullary carcinoma of thyroid (caused by reactive fibrosis and calcification around amyloid deposits.

2.1.4 D/D ON THE BASIS OF ECHOGENICITY OF THYROID NODULES

I. Hypoechoic:
- Can be both benign or malignant
- Most thyroid cancers are hypoechoic, however, few benign nodules can also be hypoechoic

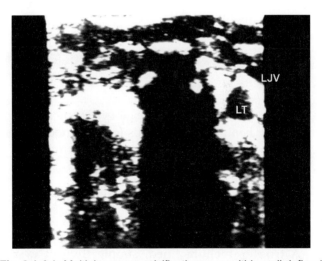

Fig. 2.1.4.1: Multiple coarse calcification seen within well defined regular isoechoic, nodule in thyroid—multinodular goiter

- Because of much greater incidence of benign thyroid nodules, as compared to thyroid cancer, in fact most hypoechoic thyroid nodules are thought to be benign unless proved otherwise. However sonographically strong suspicion of malignancy be kept
- Look for after features like-Margins, Halo pattern of calcification, color flow pattern to differentiate benign from malignant nodule.

II. Hyperechoic: A predominantly hyperechoic nodule is more likely to be benign.

III. Isoechoic nodule: (visible because of peripheral sonolucent rim) has an intermediate risk of malignancy (16% to 84%). Again, look for other sonographic features favoring benign or malignant nodules.

2.1.5 CYSTIC THYROID NODULE

Benign

- A nodule that has a significant cystic component is usually benign adenomatous (colloid) nodule, that has undergone degeneration or hemorrhage. Features favoring are:
  - Purely anechoic
  - Echogenic fluid or moving fluid-fluid level
  - Bright echogenic foci with comet tail artefect
  - Thin septations; avascular on Doppler study.
- A true epithelium lined, simple thyroid cyst is extremely rare.

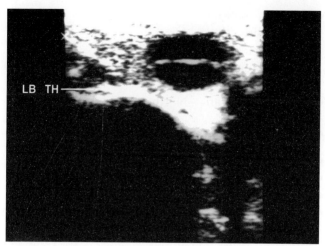

Fig. 2.1.5.1: Well defined regular predominantly cystic nodule with septation seen within left lobe of thyroid—multinodular goiter

Malignant

- Papillary carcinomas may show cystic component, features favoring Papillary carcinoma are:
  - Solid projection (1 cm or more) with blood flow on colour Doppler.
  - Presence of microcalcification.

2.2 SALIVARY GLAND

2.2.1 ENLARGEMENT OF SALIVARY GLAND

Hypertrophy

- Enlarged gland with normal size, shape and echotexture

- May be due to
  - Obesity
  - Diabetes
  - Liver cirrhosis
  - Uremia
- Racial (Egyptians—North Africans).

Acute Sialadenitis

- Probe tenderness
- Enlarged gland
- Hypoechoic slightly heterogenous echotexture
- Small echopoor areas may be observed inside the gland due to microabscesses.

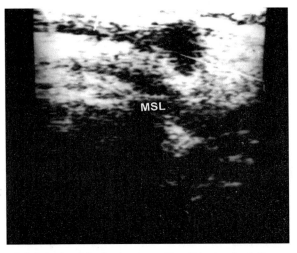

Fig. 2.2.1.1: Longitudinal scan—Parotid gland of the same patient shows hypoechoic abscess with a track seen anterior of muscle plane

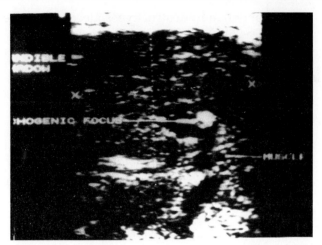

Fig. 2.2.1.2: Transverse scan of the submandibular gland shows diffusely hypoechoic and coarse echo texture of the gland parenchyma with irregularity of the margins. The finding suggestive of sialadenitis. An echogenic focus (calcification) was seen within glandular parenchyma

- Large abscesses may develop which are seen as fluid filled areas with irregular borders and internal debris.

Chronic Sialadenitis

- Commonly due to Sjögren's syndrome
- Classical triad of:
  - Keratoconjuctivitis sicca
  - Xerostomia
  - Autoimmune disorders most commonly rheumatoid arthritis.
- Typical USG features of multiple cystic areas scattered throughout the salivary glands as a result

of peripheral non-obstructive sialectasis. These cystic areas has well defined but irregular margins.

- Four point USG scale:

Grade 0-No parenchymal changes

1. Occasional microcysts (< 2 mm in diameter) and minimal heterogenity.
2. Diffuse cysts (> 2 mm).
3. Large confluent cysts with septations (confluent masses) and a highly heterogenous structure.
4. Disappearance of parenchymal texture in atrophic glands with undefined margins and reduced volume.
   - On Doppler—a diffuse increase in paranchymal blood flow signals and decrease in arteriolar resistance.

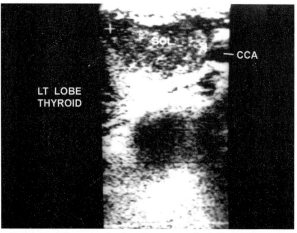

Fig. 2.2.1.3: Ultrasound showing a well defined hypoechoic lesion with mixed solid and cystic areas in right submandibular region. Benign submandibular tumor

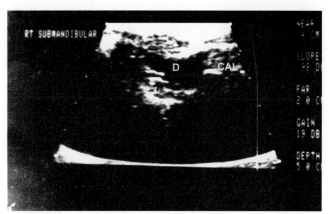

Fig. 2.2.1.4: US (sagittal scan) showing an echogenic focus with distal shadowing in Wharton's duct which is dilated. Dilated ductal system within gland can be seen very well (arrow)

5. Sialolithiasis:
   - Most common in submandibular gland
   - Seen as highly echogenic foci with posterior acoustic shadowing
   - Associated ductal dilatation may be seen.

6. Tumors
   - Most common tumor of salivary glands is pleomorphic adenoma (mixed tumor—60-70%)
   - On USG—homogenous, solid, echo-poor structure, sharp margins with discrete posterior acoustic enhancement
   - Surface may be lobulated
   - Peripheral echopoor areas may be observed due to hemorrhage or cystic degeneration
   - On color Doppler peripheral "basket pattern" of flow seen.

- Most common salivary gland tumor to have calcifications and ossifications within the tumor matrix.

Adenolymphoma (Warthin's tumor)

- Most common lesion to occur as multifocal unilateral and bilateral disease
- On USG—echopoor with sharp margins, but appear less homogenous than pleomorphic adenoma
- One or more cystic areas that produce a well defined posterior acoustic enhancement.

Mucoepidermoid Carcinoma

- Most common salivary gland malignancy
- Heterogenously hypoechoic with ill defined margins
- Marked tendency to spread into adjacent structures
- Cystic areas may be present and rarely focal calcification may be seen.

2.3 NECK MASSES

Congenital Lesions

Branchial Cyst

- Not generally evident at birth, but during childhood
- In anterior triangle of neck along the anterior margin of sternocleidomastoid muscle.

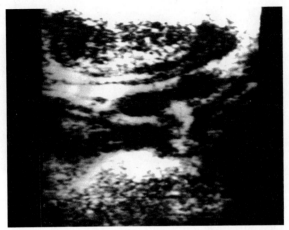

Fig. 2.3.1: Well defined, encapsulated thick walled space occupying lesion seen in anterior triangle of neck in lower half. The contents of the lesion were hyperechoic along with debris—brachial cyst

- Round or oval, usually echofree masses with thin regular walls, clearly demarcated from the sternocleidomastoid muscle.
- If infected—low level internal echos may be seen.

Thyroglossal Cyst

- Usually present in childhood
- Characterstic medial location
- May be anterior or posterior to hyoid bone or within the bone itself
- Movement towards the oral cavity during swallowing or tongue protrusion
- USG appearance is similar to bronchial cyst except for midline location anywhere between the thyroid isthmus and the blind foramen of the tongue.

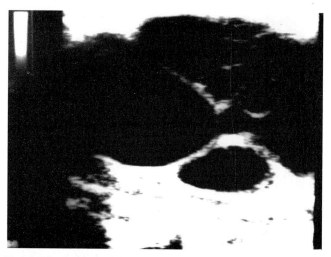

Fig. 2.3.2: Cystic lymphangioma: ultrasound of left side of neck showing a well defined multiloculated lesion with posterior acoustic enhancement

Cystic Hygroma

- Usually located in posterior triangle of neck
- Present at birth.
    On USG—multilocular, thin septa, thin regular margins, clear demarcation from surrounding structures.
- Fine low to medium level internal echos are present.

Inflammatory Lesions (Cervical Phlegmon and Abscess)

- Usually involve the subcutaneous and subfascial planes but may extend into deeper structures.

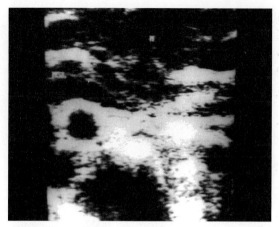

Fig. 2.3.3: Multiple tubercular abscess—a transverse sonogram in a patient of hypoechoic ill defined mass within the strap muscles—tubercular etiology

- On USG—echofree or echo-poor fluid collection with thick irregular wall with irregular margins extending through fascial and muscular planes
- Always associated with local adenopathy.
- May cause thrombosis of the internal jugular chain.

Benign Tumors

Hemangioma

- Can be either cutaneous or deeply located
- Soft, relatively mobile, sometimes pulsatile masses. USG—mass of low reflectivity with irregular margins
- May show tubular hypoechoic areas or sponge like pattern due to tiny vessels and/or small blood pools.

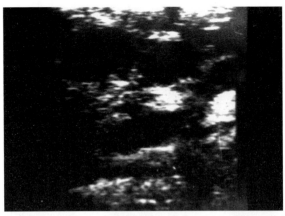

Fig. 2.3.4: Multiple matted lymph nodes seen. All multiple abscesses regressed on ATT

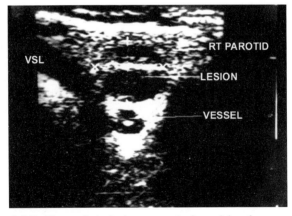

Fig. 2.3.5: Hypoechoic lesion seem to be arising from parotid and reaching upto submandibular gland. Vessels were seen reaching upto margin of the lesions

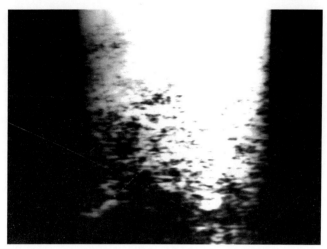

Fig. 2.3.6: Ultrasound, neck showing homogenously hyper-echoic lesion containing linear echogenic lines parallel to skin surface—lipoma

- Phleboliths may be seen as echogenic foci with posterior acoustic shadowing
- Internal flow may be seen on Doppler.

Lipoma

- Either subcutaneous or in deep tissue spaces
- May be well circumscribed or diffuse
  USG—moderately or highly reflective encapsulated masses with fibrous strands
- No signs of local invasion, with well defined margins
- No flow signals on Doppler studies.

Nerve Tumors

(Ganglioneuromas, neurinomas (schwannomas and neurofibromas)

- Their typical site along the nerve paths and atrophy of the adjacent muscular structures supplied by them.

     USG—Homogenous masses of low reflectivity with regular margins, often surrounded by highly reflective rim.
- Adjacent structures are generally displaced and compressed, but are never invaded by the mass
- Show little or no internal flow, except for carotid body tumors (chemodectomas) which have characterstic location at cervical vessels and are highly vascular.

Malignant Tumors

- Except for thyroid cancer, malignant cervical neoplasms are rare—can be
  - Branchial epithelioma
  - Malignant chemodectoma
  - Liposarcoma
  - Rhabdomyosarcoma—tumors of cervical esophagus.
- USG—Signs s/o malignancy are:
  - Lobulated, irregular-ill defined margins
  - Invasion or infiltration of adjacent muscles or blood vessels.
  - No distinguishing feature for individual malignancy.
- Tumors arising from pharynx or esophagus can be shown to have relationship with digestive tract on ultrasound or barium studies.

2.4 CERVICAL LYMPHADENOPATHY

Features of cervical lymphadenopathy

	Features	*Benign*	*Malignant*
1.	Roundness index (L > S) Long /short axis diameter	-> 2	< 2
2.	Hilum present	Echogenic hilum (slit like) or eccenteric hilum or completely absent	Thin hilum
3.	Eccenteric cortical widening	Less common	More common
4.	Pattern of involvement	Usually diffuse cortical involvement	Usually multifocal
5.	Flow pattern	Completely absent limited to hilar region	Diffuse increase in vascularity, with a wide range of velocities and uneven distribution mainly concentrated in the cortex.
6.	Extracapsular nodal spread	Usually absent	Present more often

Some Characteristic Ultrasound Appearances

- In lymphomas (untreated) the node is usually markedly echo poor (pseudocystic) owing to the homogenous arrangement of cellular sheets

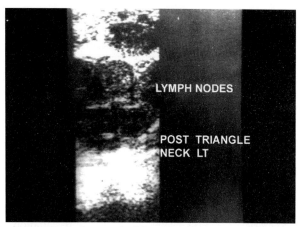

Fig. 2.4.1: Posterior cervical lymph nodes were also enlarged and showed evidence of cavitation, matting and distal enhancement suggestive of tubercular etiology

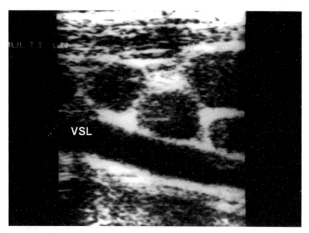

Fig. 2.4.2: Multiple large size, discrete, hypoechoic, supraclavicular (Region-7) nodes seen. No distal enhancement, matting, of envolvement of surrounding soft tissues—Metastatic lymph nodes—abdominal scanning revealed gallbladder malignancy

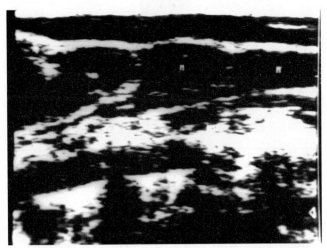

Fig. 2.4.3: Multiple hypoechoic discrete lymph nodes in submandibular region, (Region-2) without matting of involvement of surrounding tissues alongwith distal enhancement. FNAC—lymphomatous changes

- Cystic cervical nodes may be seen in metastatic deposits from squamous cell carcinoma or cystic papillary carcinoma of the thyroid gland
- Large cortical calcification may occur in granulomatous diseases or in metastatic muscles following radiotherapy or chemotherapy
- Microcalcification may occurs in nodes, following metastasis from papillary or medullary carcinomas of the thyroid gland.

3

Hepatobiliary System and Abdomen

D/D OF LIVER LESIONS

3.1 GENERALIZED INCREASED IN LIVER ECHOGENICITY

1. Fatty infiltration
2. Cirrhosis
3. Hepatitis

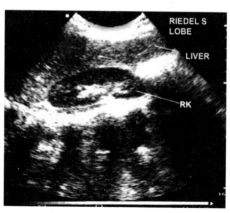

Fig. 3.1.1: Riedel's lobe—it is an extension (inferior) of the right lobe which often overlies the kidney

  i. Acute alcoholic hepatitis.
 ii. Chronic hepatitis.
iii. Granulomatous hepatitis.

Fatty Infiltration

Fatty infiltration is an acquired, reversible disorder of metabolism resulting in an accumulation of triglycerides within the hepatocytes.

The MC cause of fatty liver is obesity. Other causes of fatty liver are

- Excessive alcohol intake
- Hyperlipidemia
- Diabetes
- Excessive exo or endogenous corticosteroids
- Pregnancy
- Glycogen storage disease, etc.

Sonographically liver shows, increased echogenicity with a normal smooth echotexture giving the typical appearance of a 'bright liver' increased attenuation of sound beam is also a feature here. Fatty infiltration can be divided into three categories.

1. Mild—minimal diffuse increase in echogenicity, normal visualization of diaphragm and intrahepatic vessel border.

2. Moderate—diffuse increase in echogenicity of liver, slightly impaired visualization of intrahepatic vessel border and diaphragm.

3. Severe—marked increase in echogenicity, poor penetration of posterior segment of right lobe of liver, poor or nonvisualization of hepatic vessels and diaphragm.

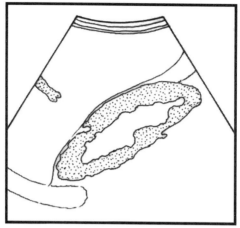

Fig. 3.1.2: Diffuse increase in echogenicity of liver—
to be compared with renal echogenicity

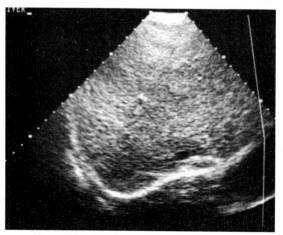

Fig. 3.1.3: Coarse echotexture of the entire liver
suggestive of diffuse infiltrative pathology

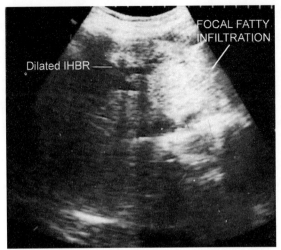

Fig. 3.1.4: Focal fatty infiltration in transverse scan of liver showing focal fatty change as hyperechoic well-defined lesion with no distortion of normal vascular architecture

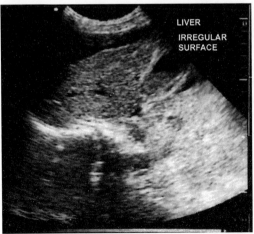

Fig. 3.1.5: Irregular liver surface is seen clearly due to ascites in a case of cirrhosis

Cirrhosis

Cirrhosis is a diffuse process characterized by fibrosis and conversion of normal liver architecture into structurally abnormal nodules.

Cirrhosis can be classifed into:
1. Micronodular—nodules are of size .1 to 1 cm.
2. Macronodular—characterized by nodules of varying sizes, upto 5 cm in diameter.

Etiology
1. Alcohal consumption—MC cause of micronodular cirrhosis.
2. Chronic viral hepatitis—MC cause of macronodular cirrhosis.
3. Biliary cirrhosis.
4. Wilson's disease.
5. Primary sclerosing cholangitis.
6. Hemochromatosis.

Sonographic findings of cirrhosis
- Volume redistribution—in early stage liver may enlarge while in advanced stage it may shrunken with relative enlargement of caudate or left or both lobes of liver. The ratio of width of caudate and right lobe of liver of more than .65 is considered indicative of cirrhosis
- Increased echogenicity with no significant increased attenuation of sound beam
- Coarse and heterogenous echotexture—loss of definition of the portal vein walls
- Nodular surface—irregularity of the liver surface as seen in micronodular disease is a definitive sign of cirrhosis.

Hepatitis

- Acute alcoholic hepatitis—an enlarged 'right' liver showing increased attenuation of sound beam is evident on ultrasonography. Clinical history is required to distinguish it from other causes of fatty infiltration.
- Regenerative nodules—represents regenerating hepatocytes surrounded by a fibrous septa. On ultrasound they appear as iso or hypo echoic with a thin echogenic border.
- Dysplastic nodules—larger than regenerating nodules, and premalignant.

Chronic hepatitis   The sonographic features are:
- Diffusely increased echogenicity and altered echotexture
- Increased attenuation may be seen depending upon the amount of fatty change

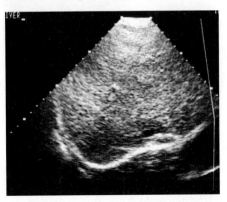

Fig. 3.1.6: Coarse and increased echotexture of liver with loss of definition portal vein wall—cirrhosis

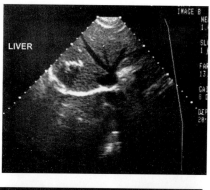

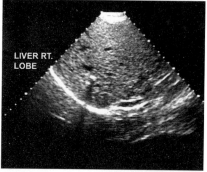

Fig. 3.1.7A and B: Healed granuloma seen in right lobe of liver as hyperechoic focus with distal acoustic shadowing

- Periportal cuffing
- Hepatomegaly
- Thickening of gallbladder wall.

Granulomatous hepatitis occurs in tuberculosis, sarcoidosis and brucellosis and may appear as a bright liver indistinguishable from other causes of increased echogenicity.

3.2 GENERALIZED DECREASE IN ECHOGENICITY OF LIVER

1. *Acute hepatitis:* In this condition there is diffuse swelling of the hepatocytes, proliferation of the Kupffer cells lining. On Ultrasound the liver appears diffusely hypoechoic and is referred is as 'dark liver.' *Other features are:*
   - Accentuated brightness of the portal triads
   - Periportal cuffing
   - Hepatomegaly and
   - Thickening of gallbladder wall.
2. *Diffuse malignant infiltration*—homogenous hypoechoic appearance is not very common. However diffuse disorganization of the hepatic parenchyma is common from. Breast, lung and malignant melanoma are the most common primary tumors to give this type of pattern. Leukemic or lymphomatous infiltration also gives this sonographic appearance.

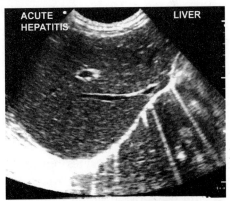

Fig. 3.2.1: Acute hepatitis

3. *Candidiasis*—most common appearance. This corresponds to progressive fibrosis.
4. *Congestive cardiac failure.*
5. *AIDS.*
6. *Radiation injury.*

3.3 SOLITARY ECHOGENIC LIVER MASS

1. Focal fatty infiltraticn
2. Fibrosis
3. Adenoma
4. Lipoma
5. Focal nodular hyperplasia
6. Hemangioma
7. Hepatoma
8. Metastasis
9. Hematoma

1. *Focal Fatty Infiltration*—regions of increased echogenicity are present within a background of normal liver parenchyma. Most common seen in the periportal region of medial segment of left lobe of liver.
   - Lack of mass effect
   - No displacement of hepatic vessels
   - Geographic margin
   - Rapid change with time
2. *Adenoma*—usually smooth solitary masses which are well encapsulated. Microscopically tumor consists of normal hepatocytes but bile ducts and Kupffer cells are absent. It is much common in women and has an association with the use of oral

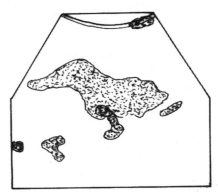

Fig. 3.3.1: The areas of increased fat content are sharply demarcated and more echogenic than the surrounding hepatic parenchyma. They can assume a geographic configuration and have no space-occccupying effect

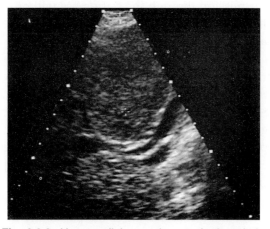

Fig. 3.3.2: Hepatocellular carcinoma: An isoechoic liver mass with ill defined margin

contraceptives. They usually presents with a palpable mass in right hypochondrium pain or hemorrhage.

Sonographically it may be hyper, hypo or isoechoic to liver parenchyma and indistinguishable from PNH.

With hemorrhage a fluid component may be seen within or around the mass.

3. *Lipoma*—are extremely rare. An association between the hepatic lipoma, renal angiomyolipoma and tuberous sclerosis.

On ultrasound appears as an echogenic mass, indistinguishable from a hemangioma, echogenic mets, or focal fat, unless the mass is large and near the diaphragm in which case differential sound transmission through the fatty mass will produce a discontinuos or broken diaphragm sign.

4. *Focal nodular hyperplasia*—is the second most common benign liver mass and formed from proliferation of normal non-neoplastic hepatocytes related to an area of vascular malformation. This lesion is more common in women of childbearing age and are clinically silent on sonography. FNH appears as a subtle liver mass which is difficult to differentiate in echogenicity from the adjacent normal liver parenchyma.

Subtle contour abnormality and displacement of vascular structures raises the possibility of FNH, the central scar appears as a hypoechoic linear or stellate area within the central portion of the mass.

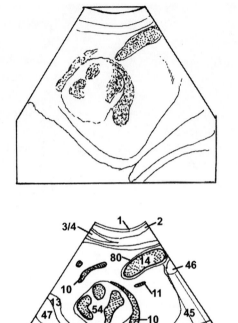

Fig. 3.3.3: Shows focal nodular hyperplasia

5. *Hemangioma*—cavernous hemangioma is the most common variety of benign liver tumor. Woman to man ratio is approximately 5:1.

On sonography the lesion appears homogenously hyperechoic. The increased echogenicity is due to numerous interfaces between the walls of

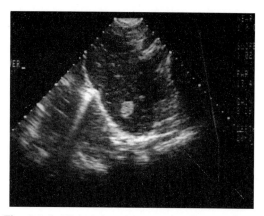

Fig. 3.3.4: Right lobe of liver shows a tiny highly reflective cavernous hemangioma

the cavernous sinuses and the blood within them. Few cases also show posterior acoustic enhancement.

Few a typical features can also be seen:
- A nonhomogenous central area containing hypoechoic portion
- An echogenic border either a thin rim or thick rind
- Scalloping of the margin of the lesion.

6. *Hepatoma*—the masses may be hyperechoic, complex or echogenic. Most small (< 5 cm) HCC are hypoechoic.

A thin peripheral hypoechoic halo which corresponds to fibrous capsule is seen most often in small HCC.

With time as the size increases masses tend to become more complex and inhomogeneous as a result of necrosis and haemorrhage.

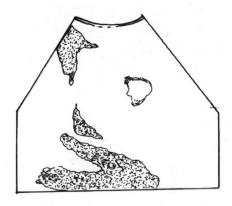

Fig. 3.3.5: Shows hepatic hemangioma

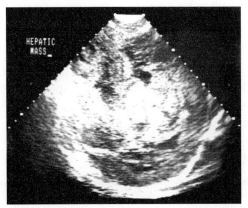

Fig. 3.3.6: A large SOL of heterogenous echotexture is seen occupying almost whole of the right lobe of liver. A rim of normal liver tissue is seen on the posteromedial aspect of the mass

Small tumours may appear diffusely hyperechoic secondary to fatty metamorphosis or sinusoidal dilatation.

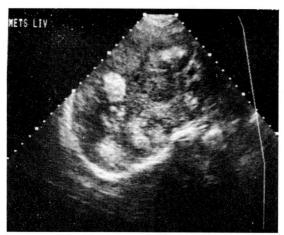

Fig. 3.3.7: The liver is studded with hyperechoic metastases from carcinoma stomach

Metastasis

It may present as a single focal lesion, although multiple lesions are more commonly encountered. Echogenic metastasis occurs with gastrointestinal malignancies, hepatocellular carcinoma and vascular tumors like renal cellcarcinoma, carcinoid, chorio carcinoma and islet cell tumors.

3.4 SHADOWING LESIONS OF LIVER

1. Multiple and small
   A. Healed granuloma-tuberculosis, histoplasmosis, and less commonly brucellosis and coccidiomycosis.
2. Curvilinear
   A. Hydatid-liver is the commonest site of hydatid diseases. The most common cause of hydatid in

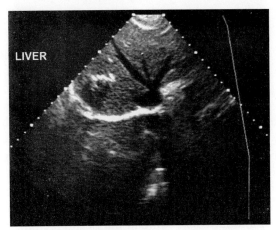

Fig. 3.4.1: Healed granuloma seen in right lobe of liver as hyperechoic focus with distal acoustic shadowing

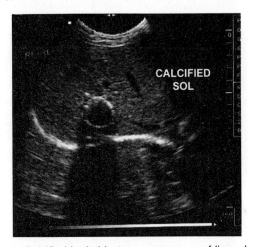

Fig. 3.4.2: Calcified hydatid—transverse scan of liver showing a well-defined rounded SOL with a hyperechoic wall and distal acoustic shadowing

human is *Echinococcus granulosus*. Most cysts are in the right lobe and are clinically silent.

Calcification seen in 20-30 percent of cases. Calcification does not indicate death of the parasite but extensive calcification indicates inactive cyst.

Calcification of the daughter cysts produces several rings of the calcification.

B. Abscess—especially amebic abscess when the right lobe is most frequently affected.

3. Localized

A. *Metastasis*—calcification in metastasis is uncommon but colloid carcinoma of the rectum, colon or stomach calcify most frequently. It may be amorphous, flaky, stippled or granular and

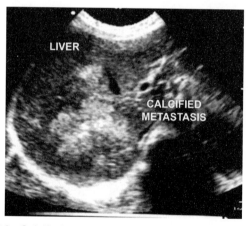

Fig. 3.4.3: Calcified metastases—multiple well-defined hyperechoic lesion with evidence of calcification within it. Patient was a case of adenocarcinoma stomach

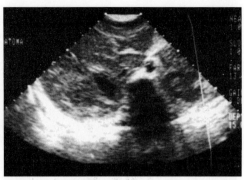

Fig. 3.4.4: An ill-defined lesion is seen in right lobe with multiple areas of hypo and hyperechogenicity suggestive of resolving hematoma in a patient of blunt abdominal trauma

  solitary or multiple. Calcification may follow radiotherapy or chemotherapy.

 B. *Hepatoma*—rare-calcification may be punctate, stiffened or grannular.

 C. *Hematoma*—previous H/O significant liver trauma may give a clue to the diagnosis.

4. Sunray spiculation

 A. *Hemangioma*—pleboliths may also occur but are uncommon.

 B. *Metastasis*—infrequently in metastasis from colloid carcinoma.

3.5 HEPATOMA BULL'S EYE OR TARGET LESION OF LIVER

It appears as echogenic center surrounded by a hypoechoic rim.

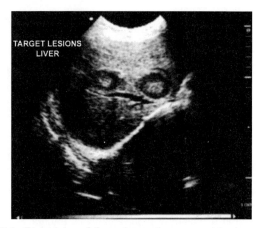

Fig. 3.5.1: Right lobe of liver shows the concentric ring pattern of the "target" or "bull's eys" lesion. This pattern is more often seen with larger lesions

1. Candidiasis
2. Metastasis
3. Lymphoma, leukemia
4. Sarcoidosis, granulomatous-tuberculosis, brucellosis
5. Septic emboli
6. Other opportunistic infection
7. Kaposi's sarcoma.

Candidiasis

The liver is frequently involved secondary to hematogenous spread of mycotic infection in other organs, most commonly lungs. Patients are usually immunocompromised.

1-4 cm lesion having a hyperechoic center and a hypoechoic rim. This appearance is seen when neutrophil counts returns to normal. The echogenic center represents inflammatory cells.

Metastasis

Bull's eye or target appearance is seen in metastasis from bronchogenic carcinoma. Characterized by a peripheral hypoechoic zone. This pattern is also seen in metastasis from gastrointestinal—colorectal, uro-genital-kidney and ovary and pancreatic carcinomas.

Lymphoma, Leukemia

Multiple hypoechoic hepatic masses are more common in primary nonHodgkin's lymphoma of the liver or lymphoma associated with AIDS.

Kaposi Sarcoma

Although frequent in patients with AIDS at autopsy is rarely diagnosed by imaging.

3.6 PERIPORTAL HYPERECHOGENICITY OF LIVER

1. Air in biliary tree.
2. Schistosomiasis.
3. Cholecystitis.
4. Recurrent pyogenic cholangitis.

Air in Biliary Tree

Could be secondarily to following sphincterotomy, following passage of a stone, patulous sphincter in the

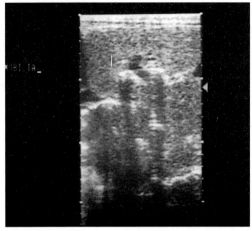

Fig. 3.6.1: Pneumobilia echogenic foci with dirty shadowing
is suggestive of gas in the lumen of biliary tree

elderly, postoperative following spontaneous biliary
fistula.

Schistosomiasis

Hepatic schistosomiasis is caused by *S. mansoni,*
S. japonicum, S. mekongi. Sonographic features of schistosomiasis are—widened echogenic portal tracts,
sometimes reaching a thickness of 2 cm.

Initially the liver size is enlarged; however as the
periportal fibrosis progresses, the liver becomes
contracted and the feature of portal hypertension
developes.

Cholecystitis

Other features of cholecystits:

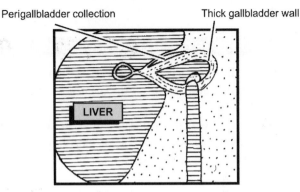

Fig. 3.6.2: Acute cholecystitis. The gallbladder wall is thickened and there is a perigallbladder collection. A gallstone is present. The gallbladder was very tender

- Gallstone
- Focally tender gallbladder
- Impacted gallstone
- GB sludge
- Diffuse wall thickening.

Recurrent Pyogenic Cholangitis (RPC)

The RPC occurs in any patient with prolonged bile stasis. Intrahepatic biliary calculi are very common in RPC. The stones are usually multiple and develop in the intra- and extrahepatic ductal system.

The lateral segment of the left lobe is the most commonly involved.

Sonography shows these stones to have a dramatic range of appearance. They can be of moderate echogenicity and lack acoustic shadowing. With very large stones acoustic shadowing frequently predominates.

NCPHT

3.7 PERIPORTAL HYPOECHOGENICITY

1. *Orthoptic liver transplant rejection* particularly seen when central and peripheral parts of the liver are affected.

    May also seen in nonrejecting liver transplants and seen because of tracking of extrahepatic fluid and severed lymphatic channel.

2. *Congestive hepatomegaly.*

3. *Blunt abdominal trauma* seen because of distended periportal lymphatics and lymphoedema associated with elevated central venous pressure following vigorous IV fluid replacement.

    Related to severity of injury and associated with a higher mortality.

4. *Cholangitis*—minimal luminal bile duct dilatation smooth or irregular wall thickening of the intra-hepatic bile ducts.

5. *Viral hepatitis.*

6. *Malignant lymphatic obstruction.*

LIVER

3.8 FOCAL HYPOECHOIC LESIONS

Benign

- Abscess
- Hydatid cyst
- Hematoma
- Cavernous hemangioma

- Complicated simple cyst
- Hepatic adenoma

Malignant

- Metastasis
- Hepatocellular carcinoma
- Lymphoma

Abscess

Candidiasis—Liver is frequently involved secondary to hematogenous spreads and patients are generally immunocompromised.

USG—There are various sonographic appearances but uniformly hypoechoic pattern is most common. Other appearances are:

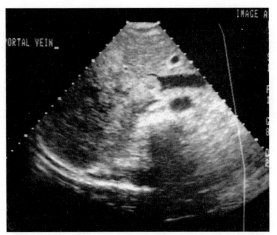

Fig. 3.8.1: An ill-defined predominantly hyperechoic SOL seen in right lobe invading the portal vein suggestive of hepatocellular carcinoma (HCC) with tumor thrombus in portal vein

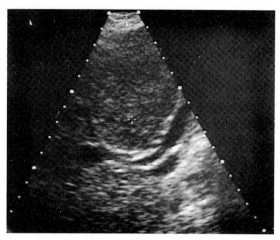

Fig. 3.8.2: Hepatocellular carcinoma: An isoechoic liver mass indenting the portal vein. The margins of the lesion are not apparent

'Wheel within a wheel'—Peripheral hypoechoic zone with an inner echogenic wheel and central hypoechoic nidus.

'Bull's eye—Small lesion having a hyperechoic center and a hypoechoic rim.

Echogenic—due to calcification representing scar formation.

Pyogenic—Regions of early suppuration may appear solid usually hypoechoic related to the presence of necrotic hepatocytes. Frankly purulent abscesses are cystic.

Amebic abscess—Usually seen as oval or round, hypoechoic lesion with a homogenous pattern of internal echoes.

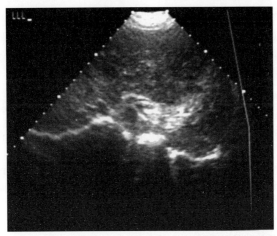

Fig. 3.8.3: Liver abscess information seen as an ill defined hypoechoic lesion in the left lobe of liver

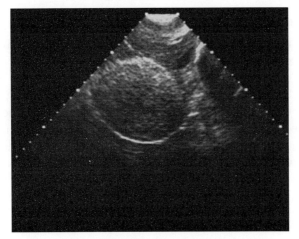

Fig. 3.8.4: Transverse scan of right lobe of liver showing an infected hydatid cyst

Complicated Cyst (Hydatid or Simple)

Following hemorrhage or infection, in a hydatid or simple cyst, it may appear sonographically as hypoechoic lesion.

Cavernous Hemangioma

- Most common benign tumor of the liver
- The spectrum of appearances on ultrasound is variable. Majority have a sharply defined, highly reflective sound tumor usually less than 2 cm in diameter and with a homogenous echopattern
- It may appear as a nonhomogenous central area containing hypoechoic portions which may appear uniformly grannular.
- A hemangioma may appear hypoechoic within the background of a fatty infiltrated liver.

Hepatic Adenoma

- Usually the patient is asymptomatic but pain may occur in the setting of bleeding or inferction in the lesion
  Usually a capsulated, solitary mass, 8-15 cm in size.
  USG—Sonographic appearance of adenoma is nonspecific. It may present as a hypoechoic, hyperechoic or isoechoic mass with hemorrhage, a fluid component may be evident within or around the mass. Hepatic adenomas may regress following cessation of the contraceptive pill.

Metastasis

Hypoechoic lesions may be produced by any type of primary tumor but they are the typical pattern seen in untreated metastatic breast or lung cancer.

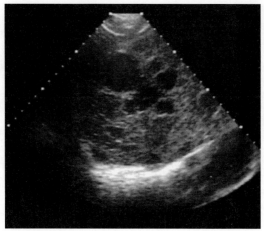

Fig. 3.8.5: Multiple hypoechoic lesions—metastatic breast

Hepatocellular Carcinoma

Three forms of the early disease are described
1. Nodular—single or multiple
2. Massive—>5 cm
3. Diffuse.
- It is the small (<5 cm) nodular type HCC which presents usually as a hypoechoic lesion
- But as the size enlarges the tumor tends to become more complex and inhomogeneous as a result of hemorrhage and necrosis.

Lymphoma

Lymphomatous involvement of the liver may manifest as hypoechoic masses. The difference in the reflectivity of the normal liver and the lesion may be very obvious, as the lymphoma have a very uniform cellular

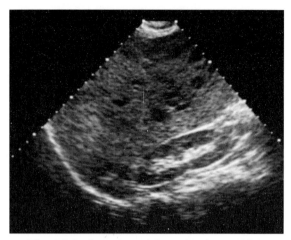

Fig. 3.8.6: An enlarged liver showing multiple hypoechoic deposits

architecture with little stromal tissue, so few interfaces are produced sometimes lesions may even be echofree.

- The pattern of multiple hypoechoic liver masses is more typical of primary nonHodgkin's lymphoma of liver or lymphoma associated with AIDS.

3.9 CYSTIC LESIONS OF LIVER

DIFFERENTIAL DIAGNOSIS

Developmental Lesions

- Hepatic cyst
- Peribiliary cysts
- Adult polycystic disease

- Bile duct hamartoma (Von Meyen Bery complex)
- Caroli disease.

Infectious Causes

- Abscess
  a. Pyogenic
  b. Amebic
- Hydatid cyst.

Neoplastic

- Biliary cyst adenoma and cystadenocarcinoma
- Metastasis
- Rarely hepatocellular carcinoma and cavernous hemangioma.

Miscellaneous

- Hematoma
- Biloma

Hepatic Cyst

The frequent presence of columnar epithelium within simple hepatic cysts suggests they have a ductal origin, although their precise cause is unclear.

- Patient is usually asymptomatic, occasionally may develop pain and fever secondary to cyst hemorrhage or infection.

  USG—Benign hepatic cysts are anechoic with a well-defined, thin wall and posterior acoustic enhancement. On hemorrhage or infection, the cyst may contain internal echoes and septations, a thickened wall or may appear solid.

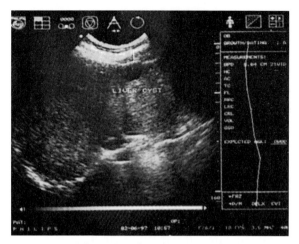

Fig. 3.9.1: Simple liver cyst

Peribiliary Cysts

These cysts have been described in patients with severe liver disease. Usually range in size from 0.2 to 2.5 cm and located centrally within the porta hepatis or at the junction of the main right and left hepatic ducts.

USG—seen as discrete, clustered cysts or as tubuler appearing structures having thin septae, paralleling the bile ducts and portal veins.

Adult Polycystic Disease

Polycystic renal disease is a relatively common condition affecting 1 in 500. Approximately one-thirds of patients with polycystic kidney disease are found to have liver cysts.

- Polycystic liver disease is more likely to be symptomatic than simple cysts

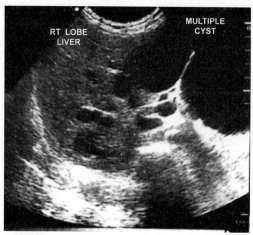

Fig. 3.9.2: Polycystic liver—multiple simple cysts of variable sizes are seen in transverse scan of adult liver in a case of polycystic kidney disease

USG—Multiple cysts may distort the liver architecture or cause hepatomegaly. As with simple cysts hemorrhage or infection may occur.

Bile Duct Hamartoma (Von Megenberg Complexes)

These are small focal developmental lesions of the liver composed of groups of dilated intrahepatic bile ducts with a collagenous stroma.

USG—They are demonstrated as small lesions of low reflectivity or areas of high reflectivity with ring down artefacts related to the cholesterol crystals with in the dilated tubules.

VMC may occur with other congenital disorders such as congenital hepatic fibrosis or polycystic kidney or liver disease.

Caroli"s Disease

It is a congenital abnormality that is most likely inherited in an autosomal recessive fashion. It can occur in focal or diffuse form and is characterized by saccular, communicating intrahepatic bile duct ectasia.

USG—It reveals multiple cystic like spaces throughout the liver substance.

Communication between the cysts and bile ducts is important to distinguish this condition from polycystic liver disease.

Extrahepatic bile ducts are usually unaffected.

Pyogenic Abscess

Most commonly arises as a complication of an intra-abdominal infection with direct portal venous spread

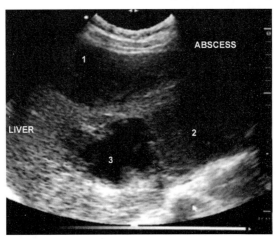

Fig. 3.9.3: Multiple liver abscess seen as large hypoechoic lesions showing internal echoes and posterior acoustic enhancement

to the liver. Clinical presentation may be variable but fever, pain, pleurisy, nausea and vomiting are all common.

USG—Frankly purulent abscesses appear cystic, with the fluid ranging from echo free to highly echogenic.

- Occasionally gas producing organisms give rise to echogenic foci with a posterior reverberation artefact
- The abscess wall can vary from well defined to irregular and thick.

Amebic Abscess

Hepatic infection by the parasitic *Entamoeba histolytica* is the most common extraintestinal manifestation of amebiasis.

Most common presenting symptom is pain

USG—Usually a round or oval shaped lesion, absence of a prominent abscess wall, hypoechogenicity, distal acoustic enhancement, fine low level echoes and contiguity with the diaphragm.

As compared to pyogenic liver abscess two sonographic patterns are significantly more prevalent in amobic abscess—round or oval shape and hypo-echoic appearance with fine internal echoes at high gain.

Hydatid Disease

The most common cause of hydatid disease in humans is infestation by the parasite *Echinococcus granulosus*. It is most prevalent in sheep and cattle of raising countries like India. These slow growing cysts have three layers:

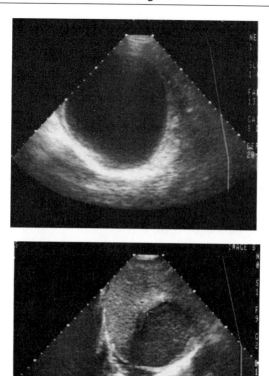

Figs 3.9.4A and B: (A) A large amebic abscess seen replacing the right of liver. It has well-defined walls and absence of internal echoes, distal acoustic enhancement is present (B) amebic liver absecess—a hypoechoic SOL is seen in the posterosuperior aspect of liver with evidence of posterior enhancement. It is extending into subdiaphragmatic space

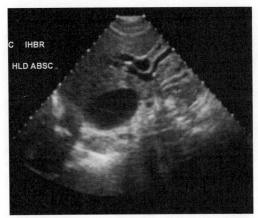

Fig. 3.9.4C: An oval well-defined anechoic cystic lesion in posterior aspect of right lobe suggestive of amebic liver abscess

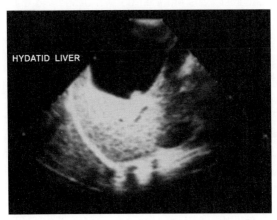

Fig. 3.9.5: Subcostal scan of liver shows a large cyst with a small mural nodule. Complement fixation test revealed hydatid cyst

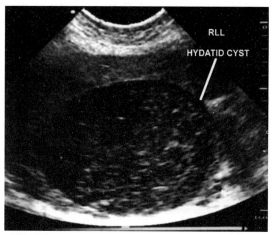

Fig. 3.9.6: Infected hydatid is seen as well-defined hypoechoic SOL—daughter cysts are filled up with debris and margins of cysts are indistinct

Pericyst—outermost, formed of hosts dense connective tissue capsule.

Ectocyst—external membrane of cyst, approximately 1 mm thick, which may calcify.

Endocyst—inner germinal layer gives rise to blood capsules that enlarge to form protoscoliosis.

USG—A variety of ultrasound appearances may be demonstrated by hydatid cysts.

- Simple cysts containing no internal architecture except sand, visibility of this can be improved by moving the patient during examination
- Separation of the membrane producing a pathognomonic 'ultrasound" waterlily sign' results from detachment and collapse of the inner germinal layer from the ectocyst

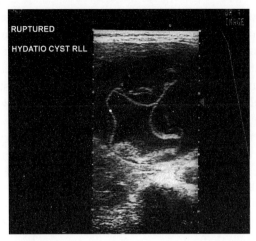

Fig. 3.9.7: Hydatid cyst in a liver showing complete detachment of membranes giving the pathognomic appearance of ultrasound waterlily sign. Hydatid sand is also seen at the bottom of the cyst

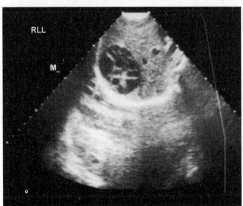

Fig. 3.9.8: Classical hydatid cyst: pathognomic appearance of hydatid cyst with multiple daughter cyst producing the characteristic cart wheel or honeycomb appearance

- Daughter cysts—the development of daugher cysts from the lining germinal membrane produces a characteristic appearance of cysts enclosed with a cyst, described as a cart wheel or honeycomb cyst
- Multiple cysts—with heavy or continued infestation multiple primary parent cysts may develop with in the liver, often producing hepatomegaly with normal liver tissue between the individual cysts.

Densely calcified masses—The distinction between simple cyst and hydatid disease of simple type may be aided by following features:

- Wall calcification may occur after many years in hydatid after the initial infection. Simple liver cysts rarely calcify
- Debris consisting of sand or scoliosis may be present within hydatid cysts.

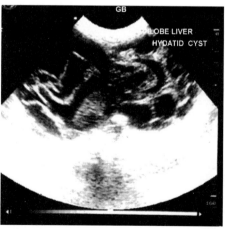

Fig. 3.9.9: Two adjacent hydatid cysts, one showing detachment of germinal layer and the other showing multiple daughter cysts

- It may be possible to discern the two layers of the wall of a hydatid cyst.

Biliary Cystadenoma and Cystadenocarcinoma

Biliary cystadenoma are rare, usually slow growing multilocular cystic masses, more commonly seen in Rt lobe of liver. They occur predominantly in middle aged woman and are considered premalignant lesions.

USG—Usually seen as a solitary cystic mass with thick septae, mural noduler and rarely capsular calcification. Polypoid, pedunculated excrescences are seen more commonly in biliary cystadenocarcinoma than in cystadenoma.

Metastasis

Mostly the cystic metastasis occurs due to extensive necrosis, seen more commonly in metastatic sarcoma,

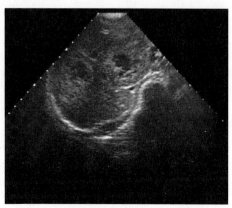

Fig. 3.9.10: Two large metastatic lesions are seen with central hypoechoic areas with irregular margins suggestive of necrosis

which typically have low level echoes and a shaggy, thickened wall.

Uncommonly primary neoplasms having a cystic component may produce cystic lesions such as colorectal carcinoma and cystadenocarcinoma of the ovary.

Cystic metastasis can be distinguished from the benign hepatic cyst by features like presence of mural nodules, thick walls, fluid-fluid levels and internal septations.

Hepatocellular Carcinoma and Giant Cavernous Hemangioma

These are the two most common primary neoplasms of the liver that rarely manifest as an entirely or partially cystic mass, usually related to internal necrosis.

In about 90 percent of patients with HCC, complications or signs of underlying liver cirrhosis, such as left hepatic lobe or caudate lobe hypertrophy, regenerating nodules, splenomegaly, etc. may be seen. Tumor characteristics of HCC like biliary or vascular invasion and a capsule should suggest the diagnosis.

Liver Hematoma

The etiology of a liver hematoma may be blunt abdominal trauma or rupture of a neoplasm such as a hepatic adenoma or cavernous hemangioma.

USG—an acute hematoma tends to be highly reflective because of fibrin and erythrocytes forming multiple acoustic interfaces. Over a period of months

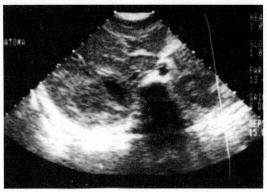

Fig. 3.9.11: An ill-defined lesion is seen in right lobe with multiple areas of hypo and hyperechogenicity suggestive of resolving hematoma in a patient of blunt abdominal trauma

the hematoma usually become cystic and develop internal septations.

3.10 MIXED CYSTIC AND SOLID LESIONS

- Complicated cyst—simple, hydatid
- Abscess
- Hepatic adenoma
- Cystadenoma and cystadenocarcinoma
- Hepatocellular carcinoma

Complicated Cyst—Simple or Hydatid

Ultrasound is the best way to confirm the cystic nature of a cystic mass. Cysts complicated by infection or hemorrhage may show solid areas, septations or internal debris.

Abscess

A developing amebic or pyogenic liver abscess may show varied appearance with frankly purulent areas appearing cystic and regions of early suppuration appearing solid.

The Abscess wall varies from well defined to irregular and thick.

Hepatic Adenoma

Sonography typically demonstrates a large hyperechoic lesion with central anechoic areas corresponding to zones of internal hemorrhage, if present. But this is not specific.

Occasionally adenomas may undergo massive necrotic and hemorrhagic changes and the ultrasound appearance is that of a complex mass with large cystic areas.

Color Doppler may identity intratumoral veins, a finding absent in focal nodular hyperplasia may be a useful differentiating feature.

Cystadenoma and Cystadenocarcinoma

Probably congenital in origin because of presence of aberrant bile ducts.

USG—appears as multiple communicating cysts with mural nodules. Papillary projections and mural calcification may also be seen.

- Combination of septation with nodularity is suggestive cystadenocarcinoma.

Hepatocellular Carcinoma

Ultrasonography can detect extremely small tumors. Small HCC's (<3 cm) often appear hypoechoic whereas tumors larger than 3 cm more often have a mosaic or mixed pattern.

- Ultrasound is also capable of demonstrating the capsule in encapsulated, which appears as a thin, hypoechoic band.

3.11 PATTERNS OF HEPATIC METASTASIS

A wide range of appearances is seen in liver metastatic disease and their overlap with non-malignant disorders inevitably results in lack of specificity.

- It is not size but the echogenicity of the lesion which determines conspicuity on sonography

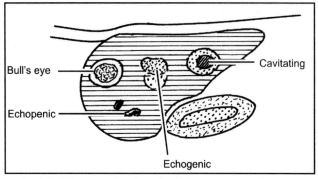

Fig. 3.11.1: Diagram showing the different types of metastatic lesions that may occur in the liver. Metastatic lesions shown are: 1. Bull's eye, 2. Echogenic, 3. Echopenic, 4. Cavitating cystic lesions may also be seen

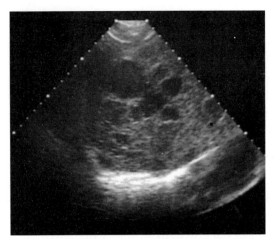

Fig. 3.11.2: Echopoor metastases are seen.
Patient from a case of breast carcinoma

- Focal lesions are the most common with commonest focal pattern of echo-poor masses.

The following patterns of metastatic disease has been discribed.

Echopoor Metastasis

These are generally hypovascular and highly cellular with internal interfaces.
- These lesions may be produced by any tumor but are typical of some of commonest malignancies like carcinoma of the breast and lung
- Lymphoma, particularly when associated with AIDS, can manifest with multiple hypoechoic deposits.

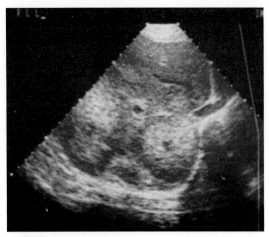

Fig. 3.11.3: Right lobe of liver shows large hyperechoic metastatic lesions. Few are showing central necrosis

Hyperechoic Metastasis

These usually arise from colon cancers and other gastrointestinal neoplasms. Vascular metastasis from islet cell tumors, carcinoid, choriocarcinoma and renal cell carcinoma tend to be echogenic as well. They are echogenic because of numerous interfaces arising from the abnormal vessels. One of the important differential diagnosis is from hemangiomas, which most commonly appear as highly reflective lesions. Although an absolutely definite differential diagnosis is not possible, hamangiomas are typically situated in a subcapsular or perivascular position, are usually solitary, measure only a few centimeters in diameter and have uniform high amplitude echoes. There are no mass effects or evidence of invasion and they lack the echopoor halo.

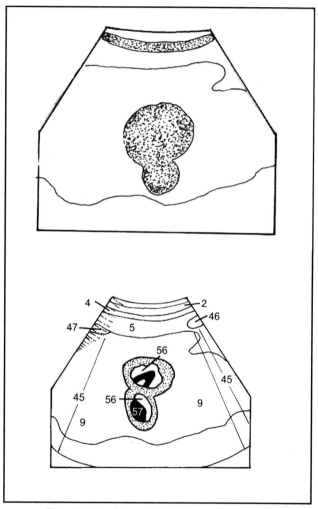

Fig. 3.11.4: Shows hyperechoic metastasis

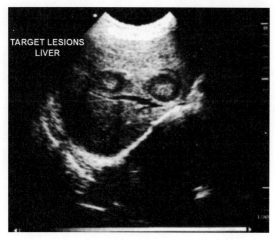

Fig. 3.11.5: "Target" or "bull's eys" seen in right lobe of liver

"Bull's Eye" or "Target" Pattern

The anechoic, thin, poorly defined halo that often surrounds solid liver metastasis is most often a result of peritumoral compression of normal parenchyma and less often a result of tumor infiltration into the surrounding parenchyma. Its presence usually indicates an aggressive tumor. This is frequently seen in metastasis from bronchogenic carcinoma.

Cystic Metastasis

These usually develop in patients with primary neoplasms that have a cystic component like cystadenocarcinoma of the pancreas and ovary and mucinous carcinoma of the colon. Usually USG reveals certain differentiating features—septa, mural nodules, debris, fluid levels and mural thickening.

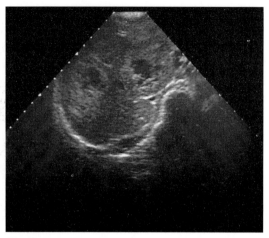

Fig. 3.11.6: Two large cystic metastatic lesions

Calcified Metastases

These are relatively distinctive because of their marked echogenicity and acoustic shadowing. Mucinous adenocarcinoma of the colon is most common cause, others are osteogenic sarcoma, chondrosarcoma, teratocarcinoma and neuroblastoma.

Diffuse Infiltration

This diffuse permeative infiltration is the most difficult sonographic pattern to appreciate because the tissue texture is diffusely inhomogeneous, without the presence of well defined mass. Diagnosis is further conpromised in the presence of cirrhosis and fatty infiltration. This type of pattern is seen in carcinoma lung and breast and malignant melanoma.

3.12 NONVISUALIZATION OF GALLBLADDER ON ULTRASOUND

1. Congental absence
2. Contracted
3. Acute cholecystitis
4. Chronic cholecystitis
5. Perforation of gallbladder
6. Gallbladder carcinoma
7. Porcelain gallbladder.

Congenital Absence

Very rare anomaly.

Physiologically Contracted GB

Ideally scanning of gallbladder should be done after an overnight fast of 8-12 hr. Physiologically contracted gallbladder appears small and thick walled.

Chronic Cholecystitis

Refer to symptomatic, but nonacute cholecystolithiasis.

USG shows gallbladder wall thickening that cannot be attributed to nonbiliary causes.

GB Perforation

Most perforations are subacute resulting in pericholecystic abscess.

Color Doppler may be useful and can show echogenic mass with internal vascularity.

GB Carcinoma

If a mass replaces the whole of the gallbladder, it can simulate the absence of GB.

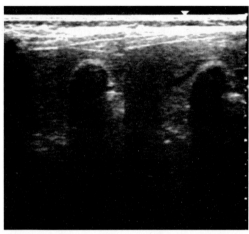

Fig. 3.12.1: WES sign—GB wall, echo from calculus with posterior acoustic shadowing are seen in the GB fossa

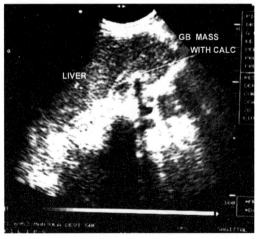

Fig. 3.12.2: The whole GB is occupied by an isoechoic mass which has a calculus embedded in it. However gallbladder wall is intact

Additional features includes gallbladder wall calcification.

- Liver metastasis
- e/o direct invasion of liver or adacent structure
- Lymphadenopathy
- Bile duct dilatation
- Cholelithiasis

Porcelaine GB calcification of the GB wall results in intense shadowing from the GB fossa region and causes visualization of gallbladder.

3.13 DIFFUSE GALLBLADDER THICKENING

When the gallbladder thickness is more than 3 mm, wall thickening appears as a relatively hypoechoic region between two echogenic lines.

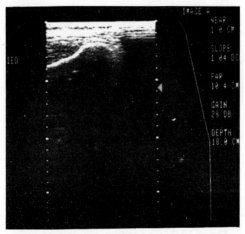

Fig. 3.13.1: Dense shadowing seen from the calcifying anterior gallbladder wall in porcelain GB

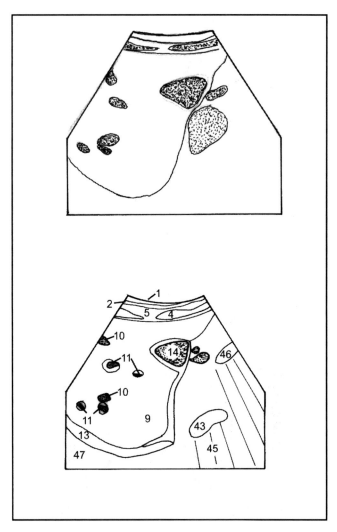

Fig. 3.13.2: Gallbladder wall thickening

1. Inflammation
2. Hepatic dysfunction
3. Congestive heart failure
4. Renal diseases, AIDS sepsis
5. Ascites
6. Leukemic infiltration of GB
7. Interleukin-2 chemotherapy
8. Gall bladder wall varices.

Inflammation

- Acute cholecystitis—USG findings
- Gallstone—infarcted at neck.
- Focally tender GB (i.e. sonographic Murphy's sign)
- Edema of wall gas in GB wall
- GB dilatation, rounded GB shape, pericholecystic fluid
- Sludge formation

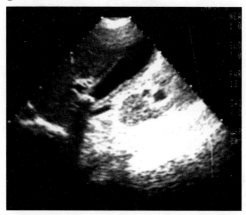

Fig. 3.13.3: Acute calculus cholecystitis—a calculus at the neck of GB is seen inside a thick walled gallbladder

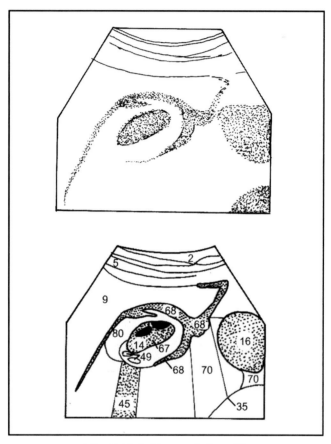

Fig. 3.13.4: Shows cholecystitis

Hepatic Dysfunction

Associated with alcoholism, hypoalbuminemia, ascites and hepatitis:

Although hepatitis causes diffuse GB wall thickening in exceptional cases there may be profound GB wall thickening with obliteration of GB lumen.

In some of these cases, paradoxic dilatation of GB with reduction in wall thickness may occur following administration of fat.

It has been shown that malignant ascites is usually associated with normal gallbladder wall thickness, whereas many benign causes are associated with an abnormal GB wall thickening.

Renal Diseases, Sepsis and Aids

Many of the patients have decreased intravascular osmotic pressure and elevated portal venous pressure.

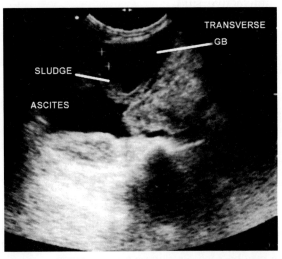

Fig. 3.13.5: Gallbladder is thickened due to ascites. Note the sludge as a debris-fluid level inside the lumen of gallbladder

Gallbladder Wall Varices

Serpentine sonolucencies transgress the gallbladder wall and extrahepatic portal vein thrombosis is present in 1/3rd of cases.

Color and duplex Doppler may show the vascularity within the GB wall.

3.14 FOCAL GALLBLADDER THICKENING

1. Gallbladder carcinoma
2. Metastatic nodules
3. Gangrenous cholecystitis
4. Polyps
5. Papillary adenoma, adenomyomatosis
6. Tumefactive sludge
7. Villous hyperplasia, cholecystitis from TB—rare

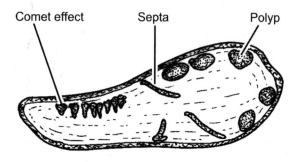

Fig. 3.14.1: Adenomyomatosis. Small stones in the gallbladder wall cause the comet effect diagnostic of adenomyomatosis. Septa may be seen. Small polyps are common

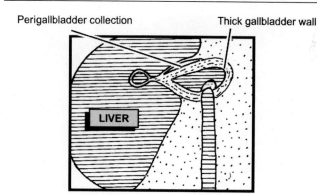

Fig. 3.14.2: Acute cholecystitis. The gallbladder wall is thickened and there is a perigallbladder collection. A gallstone is present.

Gallbladder Carcinoma

Gallbladder carcinoma can present as asymmetric gallbladder wall thickening.

Additional findings include:
- Gallbladder wall calcification
- Liver metastasis
- Invasion of adjacent liver or adjacent structure
- Abnormal bile duct dilatation
- Cholelithiasis
- Doppler examination—abnormally high arterial velocity originating from either the gallbladder wall or the mass in patients with primary malignancy.

Metastatic Nodules

Metastatic nodules are most often due to melanoma, GI and breast cancer. Less common malignancies

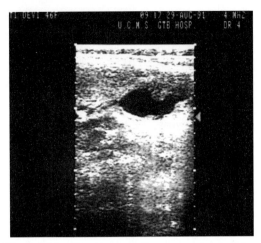

Fig. 3.14.3: Small exophytic mass seen to arise
from anterior wall of gallbladder

include carcinoid tumor and lymphoma. Metastatic
nodules often have a wide base towards the GB wall.

Complicated or Gangrenous Cholecystitis

These irregularities correspond to areas of mucosal
ulceration, haemorrhage, necrosis and or microabscess
formation.

Cholesterol Polyps

Seen as well defined focal mass along the luminal
wall of gallbladder, the base of these masses are
relatively narrow as compared to metastatic nodules.
Large polyp (>10 mm) shows aggregation of echogenic
spots on endoscopic ultrasound.

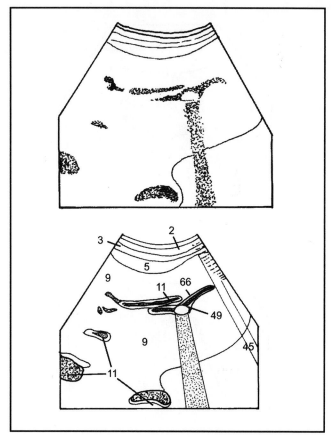

Fig. 3.14.4: Shows intrahepatic cholestasis

Adenomyomatosis

Anechoic or echogenic foci may be seen within the thickened gallbladder wall.

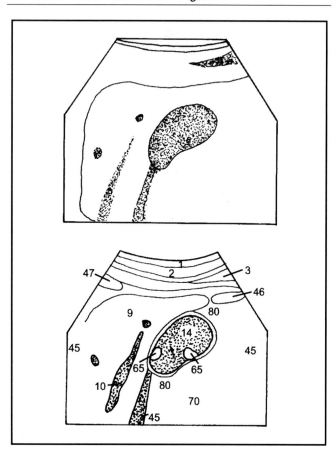

Fig. 3.14.5: Gallstone with acoustic shadowing

Tumefactive Sludge

Tumefactive sludge can simulate the gallbladder malignancy but repeat scan after few days can show disappearance of mass.

3.15 ECHOGENIC FAT IN HEPATODUODENAL LIGAMENT

Signs of pericholecystic inflammation
1. Cholecystitis
2. Perforated duodenal ulcer
3. Pancreatitis
4. Diverticulitis.

3.16 CONGENITAL BILIARY CYST

Choledochal Cyst

Cystic dilatation of the extrahepatic biliary tree with or without dilatation of intahepatic bile ducts, is an uncommon congenital anomaly of the biliary tree. It is 3-4 times more common in female than in male patients.

The classical clinical presentation is triad of pain jaundice and a palpable right upper quadrant mass.

Thodani *et al* has described 5 types of choledochal cysts.

- Type 1—accounts fo 80-90 percent of bile duct cysts. They are sudivided into three subtypes
  Type 1A—cystic dilatation of CBD
  Type 1B—focal, segmental dilatation of distal CBD
  Type 1C—fusiform dilatation of both the CHD and CBD
- Type 2 choledochal cyst—accounts for 2 percent of bile duct cysts and they are true diverticula arising from the CBD.
- Type 3 cysts—accounts for 1-5 percent of bile duct cysts.

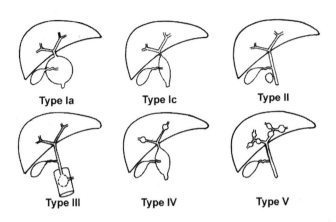

Fig. 3.16.1: Types of choledochal cyst

Defined as cystic dilatation of intraduodenal portion of the CBD are defined as choledochocele.

- Type 4 choledochal—accounts for 10 percent of bile duct cysts. Further subdivided into 2 types—
  Type 4A—has multiple intra- and extrahepatic cysts.
  Type 4B—has multiple extrahepatic cyst only
- Type 5—comprises of remainder of bile duct cysts. This type generally involves only the intrahepatic bile ducts and may be single or multiple.

When there are multiple intrahepatic bile ducts cysts, the abnormality is known as Caroli disease.

Sonography is useful for assessing the full extent of biliary ductal dilatation and for identifying the connection of cyst with the biliary tree.

The presence of stones, strictures or tumors can also be detected with sonography.

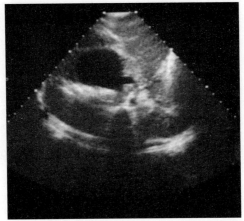

Fig. 3.16.2: A large cyst is seen in continuation with CBD in this 4 yr old female

3.17 DIFFERENTIAL DIAGNOSIS OF PERICHOLECYSTIC FLUID

1. Gallbladder perforation:
   - May be acute, subacute or chronic
   - Subacute perforation is marked by pericholecystic abscess
   - Mostly perifundic
   - Thick hypoechoic wall with cholelithiasis and septated complex fluid around is noted.
2. Pancreatitis II inflammatory fluid seeps along hepatoduodenal ligament.
3. Peptic ulcer II duodenal ligament and major fissure upto GB fossa.
4. Acalculus cholecystitis:
   - Wall thickened
   - Pericholecystic fluid
   - Subserosal edema

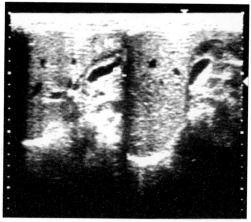

Fig. 3.17.1: Thickened gallbladder wall, pericholecystic fluid and a hypoechoic collection at the fundus is evident in this case of acute acalculus cholecystitis

- Intraluminal/mural gas
- Sloughed mucosal membranes
- Lack of response to CCK
- Cystic artery length >50 percent length of anterior GB wall.
5. Gangrenous cholecystitis.
6. Pitfalls:
   a. Folded GB.
   b. Enteric duplication cyst.

3.18 DIFFERENTIAL DIAGNOSIS OF IHBR DILATATION

1. Intrahepatic neoplasm
   - Mainly cystadenoma and cystadenocarcinoma which show like cyst with internal papillary excresences.

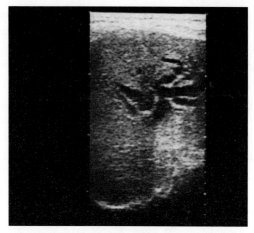

Fig. 3.18.1: Dilated intrahepatic bile ducts—stellate branching pattern seen in transvers scan

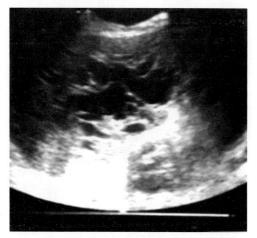

Fig. 3.18.2: Grossly dilated IHBR are seen as multiple tubular structures

- Other lesion in this category is one hilar cholangiocarcinoma also known as klatskin tumor.
2. Sclerosing and AIDS cholangitis
   - Smooth/irregular wall thickening
   - Associated with ulcerative colitis
   - Narrowed and dilated segments.
3. Intrahepatic biliary calculi
   - In recurrent pyogenic cholangitis

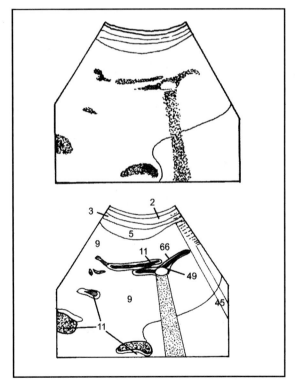

Fig. 3.18.3: Gallstone with intrahepatic dilatation

- In oriental cholangiohepatitis
- In intrahepatic pigment stone disease
- In biliary abstruction syndrome of the Chinese
- Acoustic shadows of stone may be lacking if very small.
4. Caroli's disease
   - Saccular communicating bile duct ectasias
   - May be associated with hepatic fibrosis
   - Associated with choledochal cysts, polycystic kidney disease.
5. Bile duct hamartomas.
6. Peribiliary cysts.
7. Pitfalls:
   a. Segmental bile duct dilatation.
   b. Hemobilia.
   c. Large vascular channels.

3.19 DIFFERENTIAL DIAGNOSIS OF EHBR DILATATION

1. Suprapancreatic obstruction:
   a. Primary/secondary malignancy.
   b. Lymph nodal enlargement.
   c. Parasites.
2. Postahepatic obstruction:
   a. Bile duct malignancy.
   b. Juxtaportal intrahepatic mass.
   c. Mirrizi's syndrome.
   d. Biliary parasites e.g. fasciola hepatica, clonorchis sinensis, ascaris lumbricoides.
3. Intrahepatic obstruction:

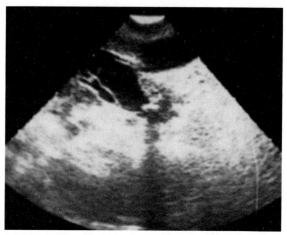

Fig. 3.19.1: CDB calculus—grossly dilated CBD (measuring 23 mm) is seen with a echogenic focus with shadowing at its distal end

    a. Choledocholithiasis
    b. Pancreatic carcinoma.
    c. Chronic pancreatitis with stricture.

3.20 ABDOMINAL WALL MASSES

Common

Abscesses

- Usually secondary to previous trauma, surgery
- Appears a loculated, hypoechoic to anechoic collections with debris with posterior acoustic enhancement

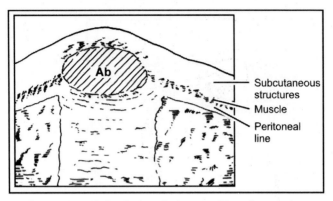

Fig. 3.20.1: Abdominal wall abscess. The abscess has expanded and broken through the tissue planes

- Occasionally, presents with thick, hypoechoic, bulky muscles in phlegmonous stage
- Septations and layering of low level echoes are characteristics.

Hematoma

- Commonly seen in rectus sheath along anterior abdominal wall
- Either post-traumatic secondary to surgery, direct trauma or sudden muscular contraction as in seizures, coughing, sneezing, etc. or may be spontaneous as in patients on anticoagulant therapy
- On US, it appears as a hypoechoic or complex mass at times with layering of low level echoes due to blood cells
- Occasionally, they may appear as fluid collections due to liquefaction or clot lysis.

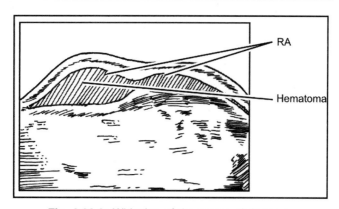

Fig. 3.20.2: Widening of the rectus abdominus muscles due to a hematoma

Hernias

- Careful sccanning with a 7.5 MHz linear array transducer can demonstrate the fascial/aponeurotic hernial defect as well as the herniated contents. (Omental fat or contents)
- Seen in cross-section, bowel loops appear as target lesions with strong reflective central echoes representing air in the lumen.
- When obstructed, they appear as tubular fluid filled structures with valvular connventes (small bowel) orHaustration, fecal matter, colon.
- CFI may be able to give diagnosis especially the strangulation of loop
- Final diagnosis of the type of hernia depends on the site and history.

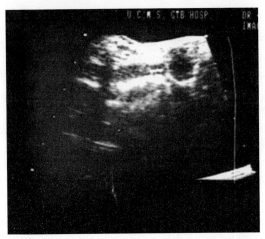

Fig. 3.20.3: Umbilical cyst—a small anechoic rounded SOL seen in the region of the umbilicus

Uncommon

Seroma

- Appears as anechoic fluid collection as the site of previous surgery
- Complicated seromas may appear as abscesses

Urachal Cyst

- Appears as an anechoic fluid collection with posterior acoustic enhancement extending from the umbilicus to the dome of bladder
- May be complicated by hemorrhage or infection (urachal abscess)
- Uncommonly, tumors may arise in the urachus in children or young adults.

Endometrioma in Cesarian Scar

- On US, they appear as well defined, unilocular or multilocular, predominantely cystic mass containing homogeneous, low level, internal echoes.
- Low level echoes may be distributed homogeneously diffusely throughout the mass or may be seen in the dependent portion producing a fluid-debris level.

Foreign Bodies

- Mainly seen due to postsurgical complication
- Most common cause is sponge, which appears as echogenic mass due to the adherent blood forming multiple interfaces.

Parasitic Infestation

- Most common is cysticercus cyst of *T. solium*
- It appears as round to oval, subcentimeter anechoic collection with well defined wall with central or eccentric speck of echogenicity.

Undescended Testicles

- Eighty percent are palpable and 20 percent are not palpable
- Of the nonpalpable testicles, 80 percent are in the inguinal canal and 20 percent are intra-abdominal.
- Undescended testes is usually smaller than the normal testes
- It usually appears ovoid with its long axis parallel to the inguinal canal

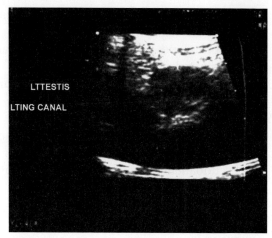

Fig. 3.20.4: Left ectopic testis lying in the inguinal canal

- Visualization of an echogenic hilum differentiates lymph node from testicle.

Vascular Masses

a. *Varices*
   i. Recanalised umbilical vein—it appears, irregular, tortuous and can be traced inferiorly. CFI can demonstrate the blood flow pattern.
   ii. Varicoceles and saphenous varices—are compressible and have typical venous Doppler characteristics.

b. *Subcutaneous arterial bypass grafts*
   - High resolution sonography is ideal in imaging subcutaneous axillofemoral and femorofemoral arterial bypass grafts.

- Postgraft complications especially seromas can be easily detected
- Thrombosis and pattern of blood flow can be demonstrated.
- Other complication as graft aneurysms can be detected.
c. *Pseudoaneurysms and AV fistulas*
  - Commonly seen as complication of catheterisation.
    - Pseudoaneurysms is a pulsatile hematoma secondary to bleeding in soft tissues, with fibrous encapsulation and a persistent communication between the vessel and fluid space.
  - Most are seen within 2 cm of the arterial injury
  - Realtime criteria of pseudoaneurysm includes echogenic swirls within a cystic cavity, expansile pulsatility, hypoechoic mass and a visible tract
  - When present, echogenic swirls are diagnostic of pseudoaneurysm.
  Doppler characteristics include arterial flow within a mass separate from the artery and to and fro flow between the artery and the mass.

Lymph Nodes

- They appear on US as hypoechoic masses with central echogenicities
- With extensive lipomatosis, they may become indistinguishable from surrounding subcutaneous tissue

- Lymphomatous nodes are extremely hypoechoic and may even be anechoic, especially in NHL with a central artery of 1 to 3 mm diameter
- Central artery is not seen in carcinomatous nodes as it is infiltrated.

Tumors

a. *Desmoid*
   - It arises from fascia or aponeurosis of muscle
   - Most common location is anterior abdominal wall
   - Usually seen in patients with previous surgery and often at the site of scar
   - Also occur in patients with familial polyposis and is associated with pregnancy.
     Females outnumbers males in the ratio of 3 : 1
   - Appears as hypoechoic masses with foci of distal acoustic shadowing due to fibrous collagenous tissue and not due to calcification.
b. *Lipomas*—appear as well encapsulated, highly echogenic masses.
c. *Rarely*—neuromas, neurofibromas may be seen.
d. *Metastasis*—most commonly metastatic melanoma
   - Other tumors that can produce metastatic subcutaneous nodules include lymphoma, Ca lung, breast, ovary, colon, etc.
   - Local metastases from malignancies of pleura, peritoneum, diaphragm or intra-abdominal organs such as the colon.
   - Most melanomas appear hypoechoic masses with enhancement through transmission.

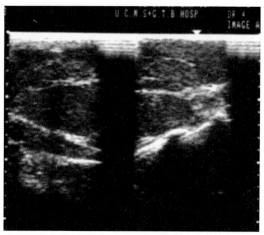

Fig. 3.20.5: Axillary scan showing predominantly hypoechoic solid mass with echogenic septae in it. FNAC revealed adipocysts—lipoma

Artefactual Masses

- Ghost artefact or split image artefact
- It arises due to the presence of extraperitoneal fat deep to linea alba and rectus abdominis muscle.
- Scanning in sagittal and oblique plane will settle the issue.

3.21 ACUTE ABDOMEN

The abdomen is divided into 9 quadrants by 2 horizontal lines and 2 vertical lines.
- Upper horizontal line is at the level of transpyloric plane
- Lower horizontal line is at the level of transtubercular plane

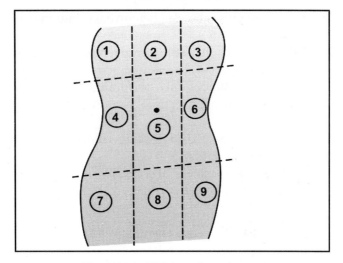

Fig. 3.21.1: Division of quadrants
1. Right hypochondrium
2. Epigastrium
3. Left hypochondrium
4. Right lumbar
5. Umbilical
6. Left lumbar
7. Right iliac
8. Hypogastrium
9. Left iliac.

- Vertical line is drawn on either side of midline through the midpoint between anterior superior iliac spine and symphysis pubis.

  The division of quadrants is as given in above figure.

D/D in Cases of Right Hypochondrial Involvement

Structures and conditions related are:

1. Liver—hepatitis, abscess, hemorrhage into cyst or tumor, etc.
2. Gallbladder—cholecystitis, empyema, cholangitis.
3. Subphrenic space—abscess.
4. Pylorus and duodenum—perforated ulcer—loculated fluid collection or free peritoneal fluid may be seen.
5. Hepatic flexure of colon—acute colitis, diverticulitis, inteussusception.
6. Right kidneys—calculi, abscess.
7. Right suprarenal—hemorrhage.

DD for Epigastrium

Structures and conditions related are:
1. Liver and subphrenic space—as above
2. Stomach and duodenum—as above
3. Transverse colon—inteussusception, diverticulitis and abscess.
4. Omentum—infarction.
5. Pancreas—pancreatitis.
6. Aorta—dissecting aneurysm.
7. Retroperitoneum—hemorrhage.

D/D for Left Hypochondrium

Strictures and conditions related are:
1. Spleen—abscess, hemorrhage (spontaneous).
2. Liver and subphrenic space as above.
3. Splenic flexure of colon—as above.
4. Tail of pancreas—as above.
5. Stomach—as above.

6. Left kidney—as above.
7. Left adrenal—as above.

D/D for Lumbar Quadrants (Right and Left)

Structures and conditions related are:
1. Ascending or descending colon—abscess, diverticulitis.
2. Right and left kidney—perinephric abscess, calculi.
3. Adjacent structures—liver, GB and appendicular conditions on right side and spleen on left side.

D/D for Umbilical Region

Structures and quadrant related are:
1. Stomach and duodenum—as above.
2. Transverse colon—as above.
3. Omentum—as above.
4. Small intestine and mesentery—intussusception, closed loop obstruction infarction.
5. Pancreas—as above.
6. Aorta—as above.
7. Retroperitoneum—as above.

DD in Right Iliac Region

Structures and conditions related are:
1. Appendix and cecum—appendicitis and abscess; typhititis and perityphlitis, cecal/appendicular perforation, cecal volvulus.
2. Terminal ileum—enteritis and perforation, inteussusception.
3. Iliopsoas—abscess.

4. Kidney—undescended or descended—as above.
5. Uterus and appendages—endometritis, salpingitis, ovarian torsion, pyosalpinx, ectopic pregnancy, abscess of broad ligament, cyst hemorrhage.
6. Urinary bladder—cystitis and urinary retention. Thickened nodular walls with debris in lumen.
7. Pelvic abscess.

D/D in Hypogastrium

Structures and conditions related are:
1. Urinary bladder—as above.
2. Small intestine—as above.
3. Sigmoid colon—sigmoiditis, diverticulitis, volvulus, abscess.
4. Uterus and appendages—as above.
5. Pelvic abscess.

D/D in Left Iliac Region

Structures and conditions related are:
1. Sigmoid colon—as above.
2. Pelvic abscess.
3. Uterus and its appendages—as above.
- *Acute hepatitis:* Liver is enlarged with normal echogenicity or diffusely decreased echogenicity with accentuated brightness of portal triads, periportal cuffing
  - Contracted gallbladder with thickened walls
- *Hepatic abscess:* Frankly purulent abscesses appear cystic with fluid ranging from echofree to highly echogenic

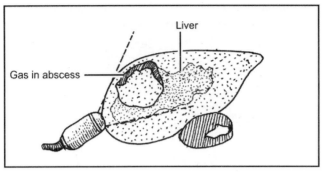

Fig. 3.21.2: Abscess in the liver with gas rising to the anterior margin, scan from a posterolateral appeoach with the patient in a supine position so the beam passes behind the gas

- Early abscesses appear solid, hypoechoic regions of altered echogenicity with posterior acoustic enhancement
- Wall may be well-defined or irregular and thick
- Fluid-fluid interfaces, internal septicus and debris may be observed
- *Hemorrhagic SOLs:* Appear as complex, heteroechoic SOL'S, at times with organised clot or fluid-debris levels
- *Acute cholecystitis:* Primary signs include gallstones, focally tender GB (sonographic Murphy's sign) and impacted gallstone
  - Secondary signs include—GB dilatation, sludge and diffuse wall thickening.
- *Colitis:* Thickened, hypoechoic bowel walls
  - Hyperemia as seen with CFI
  - Creeping fat seen as hyperechoic mass effect
  - Mesenteric adenopathy
  - Free fluid may be present.

Perigallbladder collection   Thick gallbladder wall

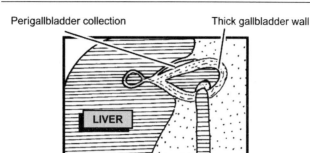

Fig. 3.21.3: Acute cholecystitis. The gallbladder wall is thickened and there is a perigallbladder collection. A gallstone is present. The gallbladder was very tender

- *Diverticulitis:* Segmental concentric thickening of gut wall with reduced echogenicity of walls reflecting muscular hypertrophy
  - Inflamed diverticulum is seen as echogenic foci within or beyond gut wall with acoustic shadowing or ring down artefact
  - Hyperechoic mass effect reflecting inflammation of pericolonic fat
  - Abscess formation seen as loculated fluid collection
  - Intramural sinus tracts seen as linear hyperechoic lesion within gut wall
  - Thickening of mesentery
  - Hypo to hyperechoic linear tracts from gut to bladder, vagina or adjacent loops signifies fistulous tracts.

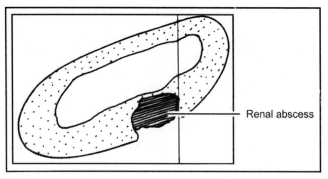

Fig. 3.21.4: Abscesses in the kidney tend to have some internal echoes and irregular walls

- *Intussusception:* Appearance of multiple concentric rings, related to the invaginating layers of telescoped bowel, seen in transverse section is pathognomonic.
- 'Hay-fork' appearance on longitudinal scans.
- Renal abscess—appear as a round thick-walled hypoechoic complex mass often with some through transmission.
  - Internal debris may be seen.
  - Gas with dirty shadowing may be seen.
  - Septations may be present.
  - May spontaneously decompress into the collecting system or perinephric space.
- *Adrenal hemorrhage*—acute hemorrhage appear as a bright echogenic mass in the adrenal bed, which becomes smaller and anechoic with time.
- With resolution, focal areas of calcification may develop.

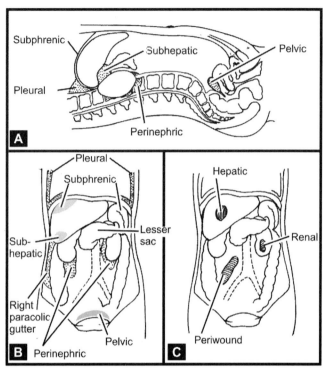

Fig. 3.21.5: A,B. A number of spaces exist in the abdomen where fluid collect. Common sites for fluid collection are the pelvic, subhepatic, paracolic gutter, and lesser sac areas. Fluid may collect around the kidneys or the pleural space. C. Sites where abscesses may form are the spaces already mentioned, as well as within the liver of kidney and around incisions

Subphrenic Abscess

Loculated fluid collection containing gas bubbles.
• Septations or debris may be present.

Omental infarction

On US, appears as a plaque or cake-like area of increased echogenicity suggesting inflamed or infiltrated fat

- Usually seen in right flank superficially with adherence of peritoneum.

Pancreatitis

Focal disease is seen as isoechoic or hypoechoic enlargement of pancreas.

- In diffuse disease, the pancreas become increasingly hypoechogenic relative to normal liver and increases in size.
- Focal hemorrhage appears as an echogenic mass
- *Retroperitoneal hemorrhage*—US appearance is variable, solid or cystic.
    - Cystic lesions may be sonolucent or echogenic with debris producing a layering effect. With time become more echogenic and show progressive with time.
- *Aortic dissection*—classical appearance of a thin membrane fluttering in the lumen at different phases of cardiac cycle.
    - CFI shows blood flow in both channels but with different rates.
- *Spleen abscess*—appearance varies from simple cystic lesion to complex or hypoechoic lesions; diagnosis made in conjunction with clinical findings.
- Frequently, gas is seen within an abscess cavity
- *Splenic hemorrhage*—may appear as echogenic or complex mass that reduces in echogenicity with time

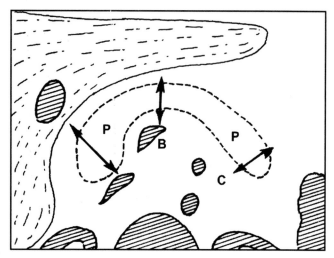

Fig. 3.21.6: In pancreatitis the pancreas swells and becomes more sonolucent than usual. The dotted lines show the normal size of the pancreas; the arrows (A,B, C) show the increase that occurs with pancreatits. The pancreas is normally considered to have an upper size limit of 1.5 cm at the level of the body and of 3 cm at the head and tail

- *Closed-loop obstruction*—US shows dilated involved segment and often the normal caliber bowel distal to the point of obstruction
- *Acute appendicitis*—US show blind ended, aperistaltic tube with gut signature measuring greater than 6 mm in diameter
  - Inflammed perienteric fat with periceacal collection and appendicolith.

Pelvic Inflammatory Disease

- *Endometritis:* Endometrium appears thickened and irregular

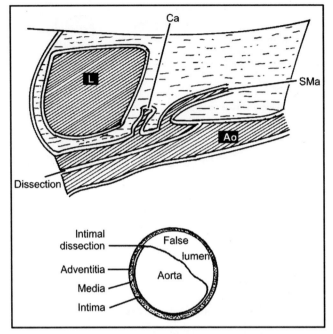

Fig. 3.21.7: Longitudinal and transverse sonographic views of a dissecting aneurysm. Note the line from the intima that represents one border of the dissection

- Fluid/Gas may or may not be present.
- Pus in cul-de-sac-appears as particulate fluid
- Periovarian inflammation—enlarged ovaries with multiple cysts and indistinct margin
- Pyosalpinx or hydrosalpinx—fluid filled tubes with or without internal debris
- Tubo-ovarian complex—fusion of the inflammed tube and ovary

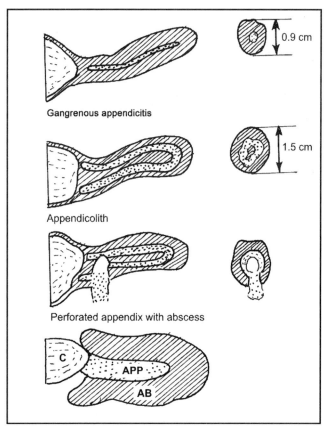

Fig. 3.21.8: Diagram showing the patterns adopted by the appendix during the various phases of development of appendicitis

- Tuboovarian abscess-complex multiloculated mass with variable septations, irregular margins and scattered internal echoes.

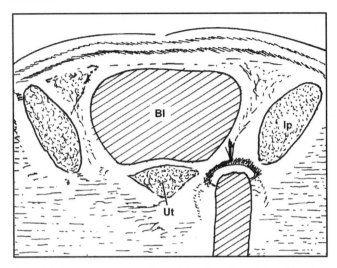

Fig. 3.21.9: A transverse view of the female pelvis with a left-sided tubo-ovarian abscess. The abscess contains air, which rises to the top and casts a strong acoustic shadow

3.22 ABDOMINAL LYMPHADENOPATHY

Benign
- oval, beam shaped
- roundness index >2 (longitudinal/ transverse ratio)
- Echogenic hilum/ present
- No eccenteric cortical thickening

Malignant
- round
- <2

- Absent or narrow

- Eccenteric cortical thickening presence

- Normal arrangement of intranodal vessels on Doppler
- On Doppler—avascular intranodal regions with displacement or distortion of intranodal vessels

Criteria for Assessing Nodal Disease

Abdominal	< 1.0 cm—normal
	> 1.0 cm, single—suspicious
	> 1.5 cm, single—abnormal
	> 1.0 cm, multiple—abnormal
Retrocrural	> 0.6 cm—abnormal
Pelvic	> 1.5 cm—abnormal.

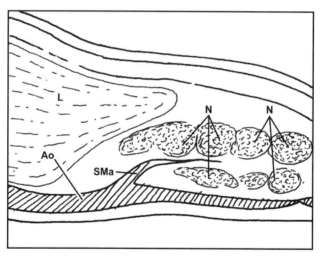

Fig. 3.22.1: The sandwich sign. Nodes lie anterior and posterior to the superior mesenteric artery and the mesenteris sheath in the mesentery

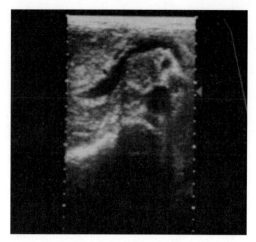

Fig. 3.22.2: A single rounded echogenic lumen seen anterior to the aorta. SMA is seen on the left side. PV is anterior to the LN. It was a metastatic LN from adenocarcinoma colon

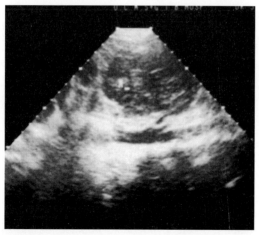

Fig. 3.22.3: Preaortic LN mass—a large well defined hypoechoic mass seen in the preaortic region in this longitudinal scan

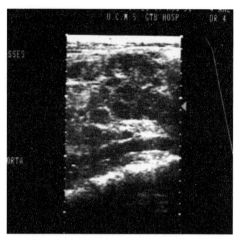

Fig. 3.22.4: Multiple hypoechoic nodular lesions with evidence of matting and necrosis suggestive of tubercular lymphadenopathy in para-aortic region

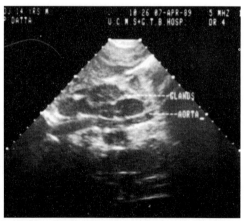

Fig. 3.22.5: Discrete hypoechoic nodular lesions seen in preaortic region suggestive of lymph nodes. FNAC revealed lymphoma

Lymphomatous Lymph Nodes

- Extremely hypoechoic or may be anechoic, with absence of posterior acoustic enhancement (helps to differentiate from cyst)
- A 1 to 3 mm central artery may be seen with in enlarged lymphomatous nodes, which is:
  - Not seen in carcinomatous nodes.
- Lymphomatous nodes may fuse to form a hypoechoic mantle of tissue, that surrounds the aorta and there may be loss of aortic outline (Sillhoute sign) and may elevate it from the spine (floating aorta sign).

4

Spleen

1. Asplenia syndrome
2. Polysplenia syndrome
3. Wandering spleen
4. Traumatic fragmentation of spleen.

Asplenia Syndrome

It is a part of the spectrum of anomalies known as visceral heterotexy.

Patients with asplenia may have bilateral right-sidedness. They may have two morphologically right lungs, midline location of liver, reversed position of abdominal aorta and IVC, anomalous pulmonary venous return, and horseshoe kidney.

In this condition absence of spleen per se causes impairment of the immune response, and such patients can present with serious infections like bacterial meningitis.

Polysplenia

It is also a part of visceral heterotexy.

Patients with polysplenia have bilateral left sidedness or a dominance of left sided over right sided body structures, they may have two morphologically left lungs, left sided azygos continuation of interrupted IVC, biliary atresia, absence of gallbladder, GIT malrotation.

Nuclear studies are the most sensitive methods for localizing the splenic tissue in this condition.

Wandering Spleen

The spleen may have a long mobile mesentery if the dorsal mesentery may fail to fuse with the posterior peritoneum.

The wandering spleen can be found in unusual location and may be mistaken for a mass.

Traumatic Fragmentation of Spleen

Traumatic fragmentation of spleen may associate with perisplenic hematoma and hemoperitoneum.

4.2 CYSTIC LESION OF SPLEEN

Like elsewhere splenic cyst appears as well defined, echofree lesions with smooth sharp borders and posterior acoustic enhancement.
1. Congenital
   • Epidermoid cyst
2. Vascular
   • Splenic laceration or fracture
   • Haematoma
   • Cystic degeneration of infarct.

3. Post-traumatic cyst.
4. Infection or inflammation
   - Pyogenic abscess
   - Microabscess
   - Granulomatous infection
   - *Pneumocystis carinii* infection
   - Parasitic cyst
   - Pancreatic pseudocyst
5. Cystic neoplasm
   - Necrotic metastasis

Epidermoid Cyst

Also known as primary congenital cysts.

Can be differentiated from post-traumatic cysts by the presence within them of an epithelial or endothelial lining.

Vascular

- Splenic laceration or fracture
  H/o of blunt abdominal trauma
     Intraparenchymal hematoma—initially inhomogeneous, later on become anechoic in appearance.
- Cystic degeneration of infarct (emboliclocal thrombosis)
     If a typical peripheral, wedge shaped echofree lesion is seen, splenic infarct is the most likely possibility.

Post-traumatic

Post-traumatic are in fact pseudocysts as they are devoid of a cellular lining. They contain low level

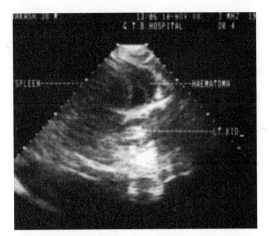

Fig. 4.2.1A: Splenic trauma—splenic laceration with hematoma

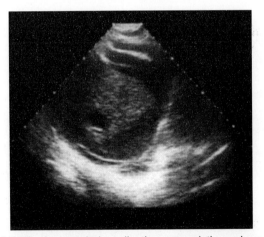

Fig. 4.2.1B: An anechoic collection around the spleen—perisplenic hematoma. There is also a parenchymal laceration with hematoma of the spleen

echoes due to cholesterol crystals or debris. The wall may show calcification.

Infection or Inflammation

- Pyogenic abscess

Causes

Hematogenous spread (75%), infarction (10%), trauma (15%) abscess may have an appearance similar to that of a simple cyst, but the diagnosis can be made in conjunction with the clinical findings.

Frequently there may be gas within an abscess cavity which will cause acoustic shadow or ring down artefacts.

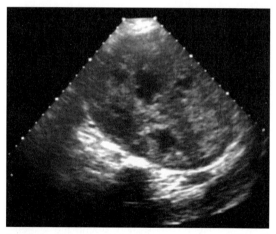

Fig. 4.2.2: A case of splenic abscess—a large SOL of hetero-genous echotexture with anechoic areas and slight posterior acoustic enhancement

- Microabscess
  Organism (esp. *Candida, Aspergillus, Cryptococcus,* etc.)

  26 percent of splenic abscess.

Splenomegaly

Multiple hypoattenuating lesion of 5-10 mm often associated with hepatic and renal involvement.

- Granulomatous infection
  Mycobacterium tuberculosis—miliary tuberculosis. Mild splenomegaly uncommon
  Mycobacterium avium intracellulare
  Marked splenomegaly seen in 20 percent

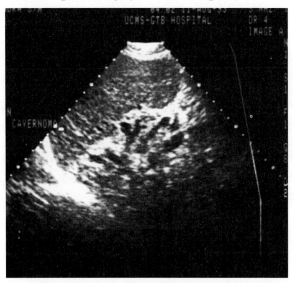

Fig. 4.2.3: A Splenomegaly with cavemous transformation of splenic vein

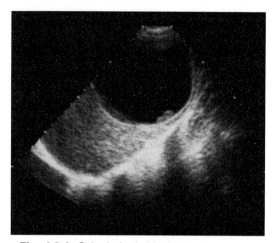

Fig. 4.2.4: Splenic hydatid—large cyst with a daughter cyst and hydatid sand

- *Pneumocystis carinii* infection—
  Splenomegaly with multiple hypoattenuating lesion
- *Parasitic cyst (Echinococcus)*
  Spleen is one of the least common sites for the development of the hydatid cyst. Calcification may be seen within the wall of the cyst.
- Pancreatic pseudocyst—extending into the spleen can be diagnosed with the associated features of pancreatitis.

Cystic Neoplasm

Necrotic metastasis of malignant melanoma, ovarian, pancreatic, endometrial, colonic, mammary carcinoma, chondrosarcoma and lymphoma.

4.3 SOLID SPLENIC LESION

Benign Lesion

- Hamartoma (splenoma)
- Hemangioma
- Sarcoidosis
- Gaucher's diseases
- Candidiasis
- Military tuberculosis
- Inflammatory psuedotumors
- Lymphangioma

Malignant Lesion

- Lymphoma
- Metastasis
- Angiosarcoma
- Malignant fibrous histiocytoma, leiomyosarcoma, fibrosarcoma.

Benign Lesions

Splenic Infarction

They are usually embolic (in IV drug abuses or atrial fibrillation) or occur spontaneously in splenomegaly due to vascular compromise. It is a feature of sickle cell disease. A well defined wedge shaped area with apex towards hilum. It is a echopoor in acute stage, later becoming heterogenous in appearance.

Hamartoma (Splenoma)

Solid/cystic splenic mass of low attenuation.

Hemangioma

Most common primary splenic tumor.

Age-20-50 yr.

May be associated with Kippel-Trenaunay-Weber syndrome—multiple hemangiomas.

Sonography

May have well defined echogenic appearance similar to liver hemangioma.

Lesions of mixed echogenicity with cystic spaces of variable sizes have also been demonstrated.

Foci of speckledsnowflake like calcification can also be seen.

Sarcoidosis

Granulomatous lesions (focal hyperechoic lesion) common in tuberculosis and histoplasmosis but rare in sarcoidosis.

Gaucher's Disease

Sonographic findings:

Splenomegaly—almost always seen

One-third patients have multiple splenic nodules—usually well defined hypoechoic lesion, but may also be irregular, hyperechoic, or of mixed echogenicity.

Candidiasis

Typical wheel within wheel appearance is seen.

The outer wheel is thought to represent a ring of fibrosis surrounding the inner echogenic wheel of

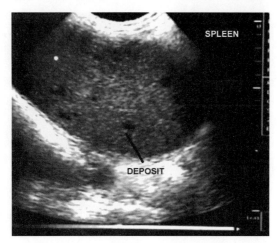

Fig. 4.3.1: Multiple hypoechoic lesions are seen in an enlarged spleen in this case of disseminated tuberculosis

inflammatory cells and a central hypoechoic necrotic area.

Miliary Tuberculosis

Innumerable tiny echogenic foci can be seen diffusely throughout the spleen in active TB, echopoor or cystic lesion representing TB abscess may be seen.

Lymphangioma may have an appearance similar to the hemangioma.

Malignant Lesion

Lymphoma

- Can be—Hodgkin's lymphoma
- Non-Hodgkin's lymphoma

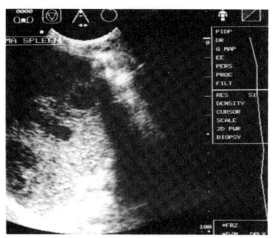

Fig. 4.3.2: Multiple echopoor SOLs seen in spleen. Similar lesions were seen in the liver and there was generalized lymphadenopathy

- Primary splenic lymphoma
  Homogenous splenomegaly (b/o diffuse infiltration of spleen)
  Miliary nodules
  Large 2-10 cm nodules in 10-25 percent cases
  Nodes in splenic hilum (50%) in NHL.

Metastasis

Metastasis seen in melanoma (6-34%) breast carcinoma (12-21%), bronchogenic carcinoma (9-18%), colon carcinoma (4%), renal carcinoma (3%), ovary (8%), prostate (6%) carcinoma.

Angiosarcoma

Incidence—rare.

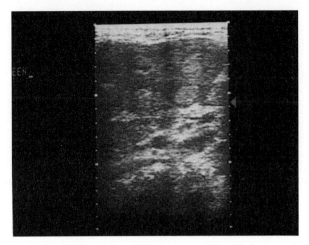

Fig. 4.3.3: Metastases. Multiple echogenic areas seen in the spleen—case of adenocarcinoma colon

Age—50 to 60 yr.

Multiple nodules of varying sizes usually enlarging the spleen.

Metastasizes to liver in approx 70 percent.

Spontaneous rupture seen in 30 percent of cases.

4.4 HYPERECHOIC SPLENIC LESION

1. Granulomas
2. Phleboliths
3. Lymphoma and leukemia
4. Myelofibrosis
5. Gamma Gandy nodules
1. Granulomas—miliary tuberculosis, histoplasmosis.
2. Phleboliths—typically having central lucency.

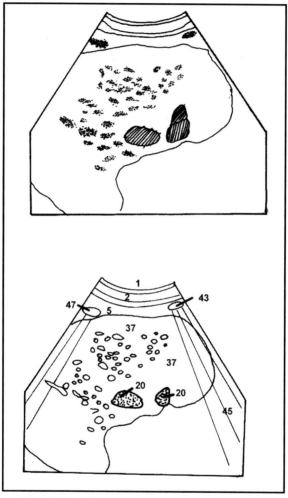

Fig. 4.4.1: Shows multiple echogenic areas—
"star-sky spleen"

3. Myelofibrosis—massive splenomegaly seen in myelofibrosis.
4. Gamma Gandy nodules—seen in portal hypertension.

Splenomegaly

Recanalization of paraumbilical vein, and other e/o portal systemic collaterals such as linorenal shunts, splenic vein varices, or ascites.

5

Pancreas

- Cystic tumors of pancreas arise from ductal epithe-luium mainly. The benign/inflammatory lesions may represent extra/intra-pancreatic collection of pancreatic juice or even areas of necrosis caused by extrasacation of such juices.

Classification

1. Benign microcystic serous cyst adenoma also known as glycogen rich cystic tumor.
2. Malignant/pre-malignant macrocystic mucinous cystadenoma/carcinoma.

   The d/d between microcystic and macrocystic tumors is very important.

Microcystic	*Macrocystic*
1. Female equal male	Female more than male.
2. Old	Young
3. Head	Body and tail
4. Numerus cysts > 6	Few < 6
5. Small cysts < 2 cm	Large >2 cm

6. Benign	Malignant/premalignant
7. Central sunburst calcification in the fibrotic scar	Peripheral calcification
8. No internal nodule	Papillary projection in cavity may be present
9. Serous glycogen rich content	Mucin rich content present
10. May even appear heterogenous solid or spongy mass on USG	Has many USG appearances a. Cyst with debris b. Cyst with solid c. Clear cyst d. Totally solid
11. Nonobstruction	Obstuctive

3. Intraductal papillary tumors
   - Large, well defined
   - Intraductal in origin
   - Young age; black; females
   - May have solid component
   - Calcification may be present
   - Low grade malignancy
   - May send cystic secondaries.
4. Cystic change in any other lesion
   - Cystic teratomas
   - Islet cell tumor (described in solid tumors)
   - Lymphoma (described in solid tumors)

- Adenocarcinoma (described in solid tumors)
- Sarcomas.

5. Simple cysts and congenital cysts in conditions like von Hippel Lindau disease
   - Develope from embryonal ductal remanants.
   - Are usually uncomplicated in nature.
   - May/may not have an echogenic lining of ductal epithelium.

6. Retention cyst
   - Any condition causing obstruction of large or small ducts leads to formation of small cysts of multiple sizes due to pooling of fluid in ducts.

7. Pseudocyst
   - Appears as a cystic collection associated with changes of pancreatitis in any part of abdomen or intra-abdominal.

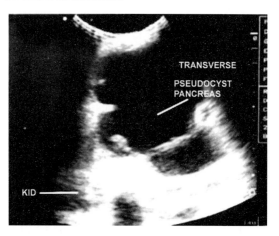

Fig. 5.1.1: Pseudocyst pancreas—a large multiloculated collection seen in lesser sac with evidence of debris in it

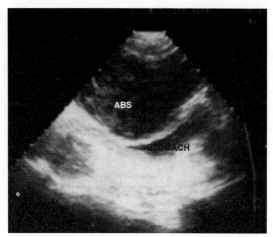

Fig. 5.1.2: Transverse and longitudinal scans of epigastrium show a large, well-defined rounded SOL with internal contents and posterior enhancement in the lesser sac

- Internal debris, gas or thickened wall may be seen due to secondary infection or intervention.
8. Mucinous ductal ectasia
    - Old; men, heavy smokers
    - Mainly head of pancreas
    - Viscid secretions fill up the ducts leading to their dilatation, pancreatitis like symptoms and pathology
    - Patients of cystic fibrosis have similar sonology.
9. Lymphangioma
    - Multicystic lesion
    - Diagnosis always pathological.
10. Hemangioma
11. Cavernous transformation of portal vein

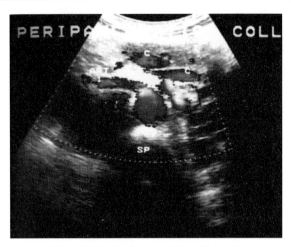

Fig. 5.1.3: Peripancreatic collaterals

- Characterized by multiple, tortuous serpentine, cystic lesions in portal, periportal and head of pancreas areas
- Diagnosis helped by color Doppler examination showing multidirectional flow.

12. Vascular aneurysms and pseudoaneurysm
    - Celiac artery
    - Hepatic artery
    - Superior mesentric artery
    - Splenic artery.

All are seen as cystic structures in relation to various arts of pancreas. Internal flow and pulsatality may be noted on gray scale while color doppler examination is diagnostic.

5.2 DIFFERENTIAL DIAGNOSIS OF SOLID/COMPLEX LESION

Classification

Primary

a. *Non-endocrine*
   - Adenosquamous carcinoma
   - Adenocarcinoma
   - Adenoma
   - Acinar cell tumor
   - Epithelial tumor
   - Connective tissue tumor
   - Pancreaticoblastoma
   - Inflammatory pancreatic masses
b. *Endocrine*
   - Gastrinoma.
   - Glucogenoma.
   - Insulinoma.
   - VI poma.
   - P poma.
   - Somatostatinoma.

Secondary

a. *Metastasis*
   - Rare, usually direct invasion by stomach
   - Other sites are breast, melanoma, ovary, lung
   - Multiple, small, hypoechoic lesion.
b. *Lymphoma*
   - NHL histiocytic

- May appear as a single nodule, multiple nodular lesions, infiltrative heterogenous lesion increasing the pancreatic bulk.

Adenocarcinoma

- Male; old
- Head most commonly involved, tail least common.
- 20 percent multifocal
- Appears as a hypoechoic, heterogenous mass lesion on USG having illdefined/irregular margins
- Calcification is absent
- Necrosis and formation of retention cysts is rare. There is smooth dilatation of main pancreatic duct and its side branches.

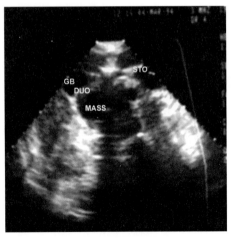

Fig. 5.2.1: A well-defined rounded hypoechoic SOL seen in the region of head of pancreas. FNAC revealed it to be a well-defferentiated adenocarcinoma

- Loss of peripancreatic planes and planes with mesenteric vessels
- Dilated PS P DV = Venous involvement
- Gastrocolic vein > 5 mm = Splenic vein involvement.

Pancreaticoblastoma

- Solid pediatric neoplasm
- Nesidioblastosis is a tumor like condition of pediatric pancreas characterized by diffuse proliferation and persistance of primitive ductal epithelium. It is associated with hypoglycemia and Beckwith-Weidmann syndrome.

Inflammatory Pancreatic Mass

- Infiltrative mass like
- Fat planes with vessels present
- Extensive perilesional fat stranding
- Moderate irregular dilatation of PD
- Smooth, gradual dilatation of CBD
- Side branches are normal.

Insulinoma

- Head more common site
- Size < 2 cm
- Single > multiple
- 10 percent malignant
- 10 percent metastasize
- Calcification rare
- Hypervascular on Doppler

Gastrinoma

- Body and tail more common
- Large size
- Multiple > solitary
- 60 percent malignant
- Sends many secondaries
- Calcification most common
- Hypovascular.

Vipoma

- Iso/hyperechoic on USG with a peripheral hypo-echoic halo
- Cystic change and calcification common
- Contour deformed
- Intraoperative USG is the gold standard
- Never do a biopsy as hormones may suddenly increase.

Nonfunctioning Islet Cell Tumors

- Benign remain abscure
- Malignant ones are large
- Calcification commoner
- Mainly in head
- More common
- Present as a mass of variable echogenicity on USG.

6

Gastrointestinal Tract

6.1 ULTRASOUND DIFFERENTIAL DIAGNOSIS OF GIT

ESOPHAGUS (ENDOSCOPIC ULTRASOUND)

Esophageal Tumors

Endoscopic ultrasound is a highly accurate modality for imaging the different layers of esophageal wall and localisation of the lesions such as:

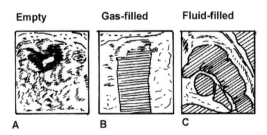

Fig. 6.1.1: Gut can have a number of different manifestations. A. when empty, there is an echo-free wall around and echogenic center. B. When gas filled there is acoustic shadowing. C. When fluid-filed, one may be able to make out the haustral markings of the colon or valvulae conniventes of the small bowel in the wall of the fluid-filled bowel

Epithelial Tumors

 i. *Esophageal carcinoma:* Seen on U/S as (a) poorly reflective tissue, (b) are homogenous when small and more disorganized, (c) when large, there is loss of appearance of gut wall with spread into different layers.
   - EUS is fairly accurate in—assessment of extent/depth of spread of tumor as well as longitudinal spread
   - Specificity of diagnosing regional nodal metastases and for diagnosing recurrence at anastomotic site.
 ii. *Papillomas:* Small squmous tumors, usually single. On U/S appears as a mars projecting into the lumen with fronded surface.
 iii. *Adenomas:* Can be pedunculated; have predilection for lower esophagus. Appears sonologically as sessile or pedunculated hypoechoic masses

Intramural Lesions

EUS has a potentially greater role in these lesions as overlying mucosa is normal.

 i. Leimyomas are the commonest intramural lesions. On U/S it is seen as a poorly, echogenic mass continuous with the layer of muscularis propria. It may bulge the lumen when large
   - Not seen below 20 yr, may be single or multiple and can calcify
 ii. Fibromas, hemangiomas, lymphangiomas are other benign intramural lesions. Hemangiomas and lymphangiomas show tortuous cytic spaces with color flow in haemangiomas.

iii. Cystic lesions—congenital foregut duplication cysts—often localised but may extend all along the esophagus.
   • Mucus retention cysts—generally smaller. Both of these appear as cystic, echofree well defined lesions beneath the mucosal layer. Duplication cysts often contain debris.

Inflammatory Conditions/Infections

Nonspecific wall thickening with preserved structure of layers.

Differentiation of Primary and Secondary Achalasia (Pseudoachlasia)

EUS aids differentiation of secondary achalasia due to malignancy by showing submucosal infiltration of gastroesophageal junction and cardia with e/o growth.

Submucosal Varices

EUS demonstrates submucosal varices that are not visible endoscopically in patients with portal hypertension and identifies azygos and hemiagygos connections.

On U/S varices are seen as dilated tortuous venous channels with color flow in submucosal region.

6.2 STOMACH

Thickening of Gastric Wall

Normal stomach wall measures 3 to 5 mm in thickness when distended.

Thickening >1 cm is usually due to malignancy.

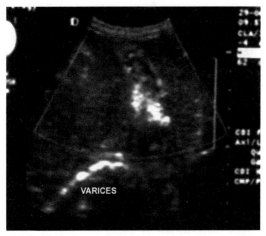

Fig. 6.2.1: Tortuous varices at gastroesophageal junction

1. *Gastric carcinoma*—initially seen as localised thickening of the inner wall with hypoechoic soft tissue lesion.

   With progression there is loss of layered structure with infiltration of muscularis propria, eventually producing circumferential thickening.
2. *Gastric lymphoma*
   • Hypoechoic wall thickening >4 cm or large hypoechoic ulcerated masses.
   • Transpyloric spread
   • Extensive lymphadenopathy.
3. *Metastases*—usually from breast and melanoma appear as hypoechoic well defined masses with ulceration which appears as bright foci with ring down artefacts. Associated ascites, gut serosal nodules, omental and peritoneal nodules may be positive.

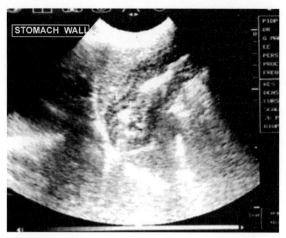

Fig. 6.2.2: Coronal scan showing thickened stomach wall in the region of the fundus in a case of carcinoma stomach

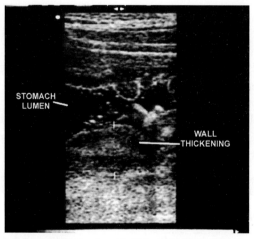

Fig. 6.2.3: Anterior and posterior wall of stomach irregularly thickened in a case of linitis plastica

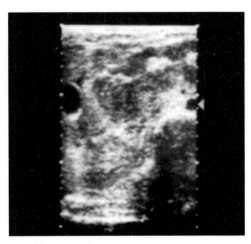

Fig. 6.2.4: A small hypoechoic lesion is seen (shown by cursor) suggestive of lymph node

4. *Menetrier's disease*—disease of adult males. There is glandular hyperplasia with marked mucosal and submucosal thickening.

   EUS aids in diagnosis by showing sparing of muscularis propria and serosal lyers.
5. *Granulomatous gastritis*—e.g. tuberculosis, syphilis, Crohn's disease, sarcoidosis and fungal infections.

   On U/S there is nonspecific thickening of the gastric wall.

6.3 GASTRIC DILATATION

Mechanical Obstruction

a. Malignancy growth involving pyrolus and antropyloric regions may cause gastric outlet obstruction.

- Duodenal, pancreatic malignancy may cause duodenal obstruction and gastric dilatation, history is shorter, H/o weight loss, hematomas.

  U/S may show polypoidal tumors growing into the lumen.

  There may be annular carcinomas with concentric thickening of the stomach.

  Extrinsic malignancies/masses may be seen involving the stomach.

b. Fibrosis secondary to ulceration, long history of dyspepsia, U/S—ulcers may be seen as echogenic foci with ring down artefacts due to entrapped air.

c. Volvulus—acutely painful condition with vomitings. Meal study as diagnostic. It may occur as an isolated lesion or combined with obstruction due to adhesive bands.

  It is often associated with congenital anomalies of the mesentry and malrotation.

  U/S may show a dilated stomach with beaking at the point of twist. Stomach appears as a spherical viscus displaced up and to the left. Distal small bowel is collapsed. There may be free fluid associated with it

d. Hypertrophic pyloric stenosis
  Adult—Infantile. Hypertrophic pyloric stenosis. Males 2-6 wk. Hypoechoic thickening of the muscle of pylorus > 3 mm, elongated pyloric canal >1.5 cm.

  Stasis of food contents in stomach for longer direction. Hyperperistasis of stomach

  Adult—Stomach wall is thickened > 1 cm with, hypoechoic wall.

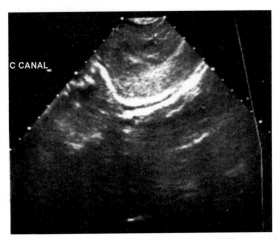

Fig. 6.3.1: Infantile hypertrophic pyloric stenosis. The total length of the canal is 24 mm. The diameter of the antrum is 15 mm. The muscle thickness is 10 mm

Extensive food residue in stomach hyper-peristatic stomach.

Proximal small bowel obstruction

Shows dilated duodenum/jejunum

Paralytic Ileus

a. Postoperative.
b. Drugs—anticholinegics.
c. Metabolic—uremia, hypokalemia.

There is aperistalsis of almost all bowel loops induding colon—with dilated bowel.

Gas in Stomach Wall

Seen as linear echogenic foci with dirty shadowing in gastric wall.

a. Interstitial gastric emphysema
1. Peptic ulcer seen as defect in mucosal layer (by EUS) or as highly reflective focus in wall.
2. Post-gastroscopy
3. Necrotising enterocolitis—On U/S dilated loops of bowel, ascites, gas in portal veins may be present.
4. Raised intragastric pressure due to gastric obstruction and distension.
b. Emphysematous gastritis
1. Due to gas forming organisms in stomach wall. There is severe pain, hematemesis.
2. Diabetes.
3. Alcohol abuse.
4. Corrosive infestion.
   U/S shows air in stomach wall as echogenic foci.

Bezoars

Masses of foreign material in the stomach as after ingestion of undigestable organic substances or hairs (Trichobezoar). US shows intraluminal density with intense distal acoustic shadowing.

6.4 DUODENUM

Dilatation of duodenum (double bubble sign) in pediatric ultrasound due to dilated stomach and duodenum.

Mechanical obstrucation

1. Bands—most frequent cause of neonatal duo-denal obstruction. Band of ladd may cause compression of duodenum

   U/S—there is linear abrupt cutt off of the dilated stomach and duodenum at the site of compression by band with distal normal or collapsed bowel. Associated with malrotation and midgut volvulus.

2. Atresia, webs, stenosis, often associated with downs syndrome, US may be able to show the cause in atresia, the distal bowel will be completely collapsed.
   • In duodenal stenosis small amount of fluid will pass into the distal bowel which may thus be visualized.

3. Annular pancreas—enlarged pancreatic head on USG with double bubble sign.

   Clinically child presents as persistent vomiting, abdominal pain, jaundice (50%).

4. Superior mesentric artery syndrome: Narrow-ing of angle between SMA and aorta to 10-22° C (Normal—45-65°, and abrupt change in caliber distal to compression.

5. Distal small bowel obstruction/volvulus.

6. Paralytic ileus particularly due to pancreatitis associated. with dilated small and large bowel.

7. Malrotation with volvulus—malrotation implies incomplete rotation of bowel. This gives rise to symptoms of associated band of Ladd and shortening of mesenteric attachments. On U/S

duodenojejunal junction is displaced medially and downward and caecum medially and upward.

Superior mesenteric vein lies medial towards left of the SMA.

There is dilatation of gut.

6.5 SMALL BOWEL AND COLON

Dilated Small Bowel

a. Mechanical obstruction—dilated large bowel US can tell the approximate level of obstruction because there is dilatation proximal to the obstruction. There is accumulation of large quantities of fluid and/or gas with hyperperistalsis.

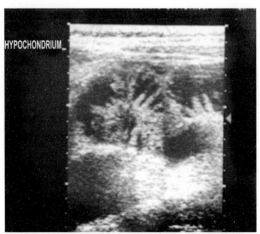

Fig. 6.5.1: Dilated fluid filled jejunal loops: Valvulae conniventes are well seen

b. *Paralytic ileus*—dilated fluid filled hypo or aperi-staltic bowel loops involving almost whole of the bowel (small and large).

c. Iatrogenic—postvagotomy and gastrectomy due to rapid emptying of stomach contents.

d. Ischemia—thickened bowel loops with free fluid, lack of colour flow on Doppler imaging.

e. Extensive small bowel resection—compensatory dilatation and thickening of folds.

Thickening of Terminal Ileum/and/or Cecum

Inflammatory/Infective

a. Tuberculosis—most common cause in Indian popu-lation. Continuity of involvement, with cecum and ascending colon can occur.

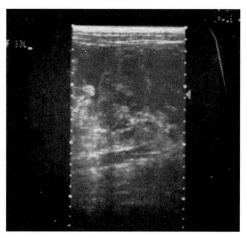

Fig. 6.5.2: Matted bowel loop: clumped small bowel loops are seen in RIF with surrounding free fluid in a case of abdominal tuberculosis

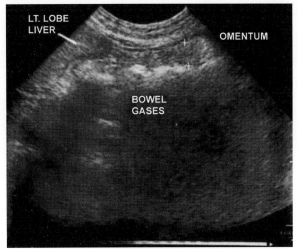

Fig. 6.5.3: Thickened omentum (1.6 cm) in a case of abdominal Koch's

Cecum is predominantly involved, associated mesentric thickening, lymph nodes, ascites, omental cake formation.

b. Amoebic typhilitis—thickening of terminal ileum and/or cecum with ameboma formation with lump in right iliac fossa. Presence of cysts of *E. histolytica* in stool.

c. Actinomycosis—very rare, predominantly cecum.

d. Crohn's disease.

e. Ulcerative colitis due to back wash ilitis.

Neoplastic

a. Lymphoma—hypoechoic wall thickening, lymph nodes ±.

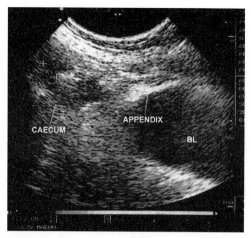

Fig. 6.5.4: Inflammatory thickening of cecum and appendix is seen in a case of typhilitis

b. Carcinoid—most ileal carcinoids originate in distal ileum, are malignant if >2 cm cecum may be involved.

c. Metastasis—malignant melanoma and lung and breast tumors are commonest sites.

d. Ischemic—acute severe pain in abdomen, non-stratified thickened bowel wall absent, barely visible color flow.

Pseudokidney Sign (Target Sign)

Normal bowel wall thickness in non distended state is 5 mm and 3 mm in distended state.when bowel is thickened there is formation of pseudo kidney sign due to central highly reflective contents and hypoechoic surrounding wall.

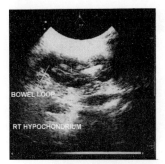
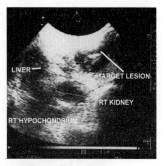

Fig. 6.5.5: Target lesion: longitudinal and transverse scan showing bowel thickening

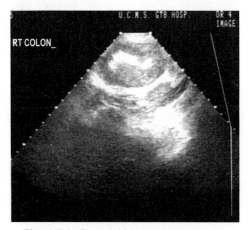

Fig. 6.5.6: Pseudokidney sign seen in a case of bowel thickening

Causes

1. *Tumors*
   a. Adenocarcinoma—most common GI malignancy, colon is a very common site.

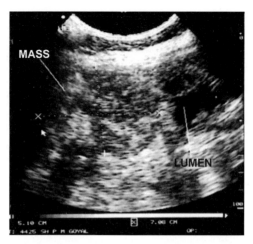

Fig. 6.5.7: Carcinoma colon—a large soft tissue mass, predominantly hypoechoic is seen arising from the hepatic flexure

It can be exophytic, annular or intraluminal. There may be symmetric or asymmetric wall thickening which is usually hypoechoic lymph nodes, metastasis may be present.

b. Lymphoma—hypoechoic wall thickening lymphadenopathy.

c. Leiomyosarcoma—mainly exophytic, outwards ulceration and cavitation is common, calcification may occur and is heterogenous in echotexture.

d. Carcinoid.

e. Metastasis—Known primary is present, other metastatic lesions.

2. *Inflammatory*

a. *Tuberculosis*—lymph nodes, mesenteric thickening ascites, etc.

b. *Crohn's disease*—ultrasonographic features are:
   1. Gut wall thickening—mostly concentric and quite marked. Involved gut appears rigid and fixed with no peristasis.
   2. Strictures—appears as linear echogenic central area within a thickened bowel loop.
   3. Creeping fat—edema and fiborosis of adjacent mesentery forms a mass which creeps over the border of abdominal gut— On U/S it appears as a hyperechoic mass effect or halo around the mesenteric border of gut. It causes separation of loops.
   4. Hyperemia—increased flow on Doppler.
   6. Inflammatory conglomerate masses formed by clumps of matted bowel, mesentery, fat and lymph node.
   7. Complex or fluid filled phlegmons or abscess may be present.
   8. Fissures in gut wall may be seen as linear echogenic areas penetrating into the wall.
c. *Diverticular disease*—segmental, concentric bowel wall thickening, echogenic foci within bowel wall due to air, localised collections, thickening of mesentery.
d. *Chronic granulomatous diseases*—e.g. syphilis, sarcoidosis, etc.
e. *Pseudomembranous colitis*—thickening of colon wall with exagerated haustra. Watery diarrhea is the most common symptom, with fever and abdominal pain.
f. *Appendicitis*—dilated (> 6 mm) tubular, non-compressible, aperistaltic blind ended structure

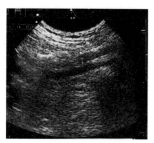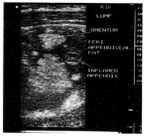

Fig. 6.5.8: Longtiudinal and transverse scans of right iliac fossa shows inflamed appendix however no periappendicular collection is seen

in right iliac fossa with localized fluid collection, probe tenderness, fever, vomitings, etc.

3. *Miscellaneous*

   a. Intussusception: Sonographic appearance of multiple concentric rings with features of intestinal obstruction.

      • Invagination of a bowel segment into the next distal segment.

        On U/S:

      a. Multiple concentric rings due to layers of invagination bowel with attenuate echogenic and hypoechoic layers may be seen.

      b. Target sign with center echogenic and thick hypoechoic wall.

      c. Longitudinal scan may show fork appearance.

        The mesentery with the mesenteric vessels seen invaginate into the mass is a specific sign.

   b. Ischemia—due to thickening of bowel wall.

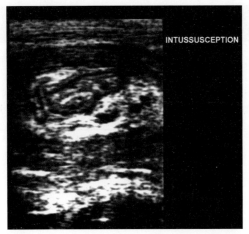

Fig. 6.5.9: Intussusception is seen as target sign—hypo-echoic solid mass with a central echogenic component

    c. Amyloidosis—pathological evidence with immunohistochemical.

    d. Radiation enteritis—H/o radiation therapy.

4. *Mimicks*

    a. Normal kidney in ectopic position—renal sinus is echogenic with surrounding kidney tissue.

    b. Multiple loops of fluid filled bowel.

    c. Ovarian dermoid due to echogenic fat and surrounding fluid which is hypoechoic.

    d. Normal colon—surrounding wall with echogenic lumen.

    e. Gas in head of pancreas.

    f. Mesenteric lymph nodes—due to echogenic fatty intum.

    g. Gallstones in thick walled gallbladder.

    h. Hemorrhage in bowel wall.

6.6 D/D OF ACUTE APPENDICITIS (APPENDICEAL LESIONS)

Acute Appendicitis

The underlying factor is obstruction of appendiceal lumen causing retention of secretions, increasing

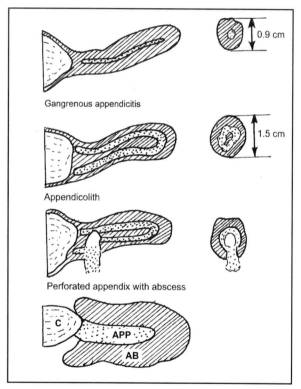

Fig. 6.6.1: Diagram showing the patterns adopted by the appendix during the various phases of development of appendicitis

intraluminal pressure—compromising venous return—hypoxia and ischemia—gangrene and perforation.

U/S

1. Blind ended, Aperistaltic tube arising from the tip of cecum with gut signature and diameter >6 mm
2. Supportive e/o—inflammed perienteric fat, pericardial collection appendicolith.

Appendiceal Perforation U/S May Show

- Loculated pericecal fluid
- Phlegmon
- Abscess
- Prominent pericecal fat
- Circumferential loss of submucosal layer of appendix.

Appendicular Lump

Inflamed appendix is encased by inflamed bowel loops, mesentery, omentum, fluid and lymph nodes.

U/S Shows

a. An ill-defined mass heterogenous in appearance with adherent hypoperistaltic thickened bowel.
b. Mesentery and omentum appear echogenic due to fat.
c. Loculated fluid collections and LN may be seen.

U/S d/d

Thickened terminal ileum shows peristalsis and is not blind ended. It is compressible.

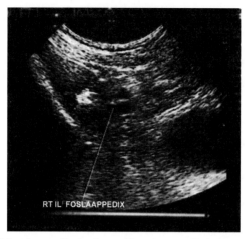

Fig. 6.6.2: Appendicular lump: Seen as an ill defined complex SOL in the right iliac fossa. Inflamed appendix, periappendiceal fat and omentum are seen in the lump, adherent bowel loops are also seen

6.7 ROLE OF RECTAL ENDOSONOGRAPHY

1. Staging of detected rectal carcinomas
   Rectal carcinoma arise from mucosal surface of the gut
   a. Tumors appear as relatively hypoechoic masses that may distort the rectal lumen.
   b. Loss of continuity of different layers of rectal wall.
   c. Surface ulceration may be seen as echogenic foci with ring down artifact.
   d. LN appears as round or oval hypoechoic masses in perirectal fat.

2. Differentiate extrinsic, intramural and mucosal lesions.
3. Anal evaluation: To show integrity of sphincters with documentation of the degree and size of muscle defects.

7

Retroperitoneum

Retroperitoneal Pathologies

- Most common manifestation of a retroperitoneal pathology is "Presence of a Mass."
- Sonographic signs apart from above that localize the mass and differentiate mass from pseudomass are:
  a. Displacement of normal structures.
  b. Direct invasion of adjacent organ.
  c. Asymmetry of normal paired structures.
  d. Silhoutting of normal structures.
  e. Loss of retroperitoneal details.

7.1 DIFFERENTIAL DIAGNOSIS OF SOLID MASSES

Lymphadenopathy

- Inferior to CT for this purpose as it is poorly reproducible and the image is degraded by gas.
- Size <1 cm = Normal
  > 1 cm, single = Suspicious abdominal nodes
  > 1 cm, multiple = Abnormal
  > 1.5 cm, single = Abnormal

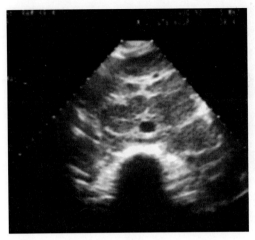

Fig. 7.1.1: Conglomerate lymph nodes mass seen in the preaortic region

> .6 cm = Abnormal-retrocrural
> 1.5 cm = Pelvic
- Signs of malignancy
  — Longitudinal to transeverse ratio
    < 2, i.e. round/oval.
  — Eccentric cortical thickening.
    Narrow/absent echogenic hilum.
    — Displaced/distorted intranodal vessels.
    — Intranodal avascular areas.
- Causes
  a. Malignant deposites—testes, GI, lung, pelvic tumors.
  b. Lymphoma
    — Multiple hypoechoic masses.

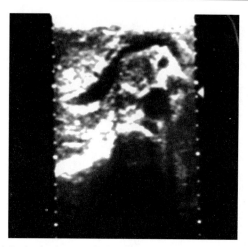

Fig. 7.1.2: A single rounded echogenic lumen seen anterior to the aorta. SMA is seen on the left side. PV is anterior to the LN. It was a metastatic LN from adenocarcinoma colon

     — may fuse to form a mantle.
     — may invade the retroperitoneum.
  c. Infections.

Primary Retroperitoneal Tumors

- Adult mainly.
- Mostly malignant.
- Mostly mesenchymal.
- More in men.
- Main lesions are:
  - a. Lipoma sarcoma—has echogenic fat.
  - b. Leomyosarcoma—hypoechoic.
  - c. Malignant fibrous histiocytoma.
  - d. Teratoma.

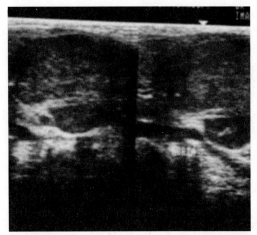

Fig. 7.1.3: A large ill-defined solid hypoechoic lesion seen anterior to the compressed aorta turned out to be a retroperitoneal sarcoma

    — Fat fluid levels
    — Calcification.
  e. Germ cell tumors.

Secondary Deposits

- Intranodal.
- Extranodal.
- Direct invasion.

Retroperitoneal Fibrosis

- Also knows as Ormond's disease.
- Causes
    — Idiopathic (68%)
    — Malignancies (8%)
      (stomach, lung, breast, colon, prostate, kidney)

— Methisergide (12%)
— Crohn's disease
— Reidel's struma
— Sclerosing cholangitis.
— Radiotherapy.
— Aneurysm leak/surgery.
— Infection.
— Urine leak.
— Hypoechoic, smooth marginated homogenous fibrous clumps are noted.
— Ureters medialy deviated.

7.2 DIFFERENTIAL DIAGNOSIS OF PSEUDOMASSES

1. Horse-shoe kidney:
   — IVP diagnostic.

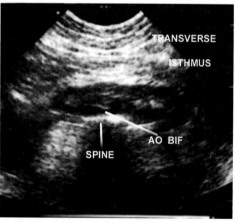

Fig. 7.2.1: Horse-shoe kidney: Transverse scan shows the isthmus connecting the lower poles of the right and left kidneys anterior to the aorta

    — Mild to moderate hydronephrosis.
2. Ptotic kidney.
3. Low lying pancreas.
4. Varix.
5. Extramedullary hematopoiesis.
6. Hematoma.
7. Duplication cyst of gut.

7.3 DIFFERENTIAL DIAGNOSIS OF CYSTIC LESIONS AND FLUID COLLECTION

1. Primary retroperitoneal cysts
2. Lymphangioma:
   - Congenital
   - Cyst with multiple thick septa or unilocular.

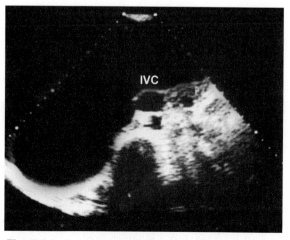

Fig. 7.3.1: A huge completely anechoic retroperitoneal cyst is seen in this transverse scan

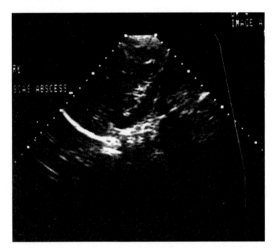

Fig. 7.3.2A: Psoas abscess—there is a hypoechoic collection in right psoas muscle

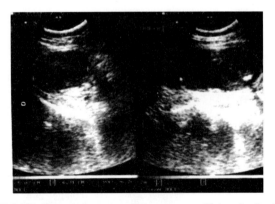

Fig. 7.3.3B: Psoas abscess—(i) transverse, (ii) longitudinal scan showing a collection in psoas muscle with evidence of internal echoes, thick posterior wall and calcification

3. Lymphoceles
   - Like simple cysts
   - Lateral to bladder within 3 cm of abdominal wall
   - Mostly post-surgical.
4. Urinoma:
   - Hypoechoic loculated collection
   - Perilesional fibrosis
   - Following obstruction, trauma, surgery.
5. Varix
6. Pancreatic pseudocyst:
   - In any space but mostly anterior pararenal space.
   - Definate evidence of pancreatitis present.
7. Hematoma/hemorrhage:
   - Due to trauma intervension, aneurysm, bleeding diasthasis, tumor bleed
   - Heterogenous fluid collection
   - Changing appearance with time.
8. Infections:
   - Psoas abscess in Pott's spine
   - Spread of infection from adjacent organ
   - Predesposed by diabetes, AIDS, trauma, surgery, alchohal.

8.1 DIFFERENTIAL DIAGNOSIS OF RENAL PSEUDOTUMOR

1. Hypertrophied column of Bertin (HCB):
   - A normal varient that occurs due to unresorption of polar parenchyma from one or both of

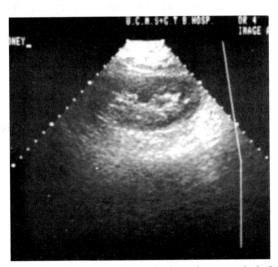

Fig. 8.1.1: Pseudotumor—the pelvicalyceal system is indented by a mass isoechoic to the cortex—hypertrophied column of Bertin

the two subkidneys that fuse to form the normal kidney
- Indentation of renal sinus lateraly
- Bordered by junctional parenchymal defects
- Location at junction of upper and middle thirds
- Continuous with renal cortex
- Contains renal pyramids
- Less than 3 cm in size.

2. Renal duplication artefacts:
   - Due to refraction of sound beam between the lower portion of spleen or liver and adjacent fat
   - Left; obese
   - Change transducer position; Scan in deep inspiration.

3. Fetal lobulations:
   - Usually persist in all pediatric kidneys but may also be seen in 51 percent of adult kidneys
   - No associated cortical loss is noted.

4. Compunsatory hypertrophy:
   a. Diffuse—in cases of contralateral nephrectomy, renal agenesis, renal hypoplasia, dysplasias, atrophy.
      - Generalized renal involvement.
   b. Focal/nodular
      - When residual island of normal tissue hypertrophy in an otherwise diseased kidney, e.g. reflux nephropathy.
      - Nodular areas of hypertrophy resembling mass lesions are seen.

5. Renal malakoplakia
   - Cortical and medullary granulomatous masses of the Hansemann's giant cells containing Michaelis-Gutmann inclusion bodies are seen

- *E. coli, Klebsiella*
- Multifocal masses, enlarging the kidney, bilateral in 50 percent.
- Masses are hypoechoic and distort the central renal sinus.

6. Xanthogranulomatous pyelonephritis:
   - A chronic suppurative renal infection leading to destruction of renal parenchyma and replacement of it with lipid laden macrophages
   - Unilateral, diffuse/segmental/focal
   - 70 percent have a staghorn calculus
   - *Proteus, E.coli*
   - Focal/Segmental varieties are difficult to differentiate from renal abscess or tumor.

7. Vascular malformations and aneurysm
   - Color doppler is the helping investigation.

8. Parasitic infection
   - Hydatid, filaria, schistosoma.

9. Fungal infection
   - *Cadida* forming fungal balls.

8.2 DIFFERENTIAL DIAGNOSIS OF CYSTIC RENAL DISEASE

- A kidney having 3-5 cysts of any kind is known as "kidney with cystic disease."

Classification (by Elkin)

Renal Cystic Dysplasia

a. Multicystic dysplastic kidney (Potter-2).

b. Focal and segmental cystic dysplasia.
c. Multiple cysts associated with lower urinary tract obstruction.
d. Hereditary and familial cystic dysplasia.

Polycystic Kidney Disease

a. PKD of young (Potter-1)
b. PKD of adult (Potter-3)

Cortical Cysts

a. Simple-serous (typical), atypical, complicated.
b. Multilocular.
c. Trisomy associated.
d. Tuberous sclerosis, von Hippel Lindau disease.

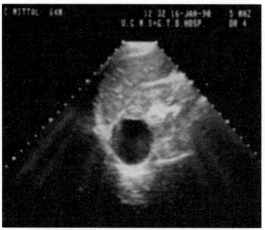

Fig. 8.2.1: Simple cortical cyst—a well defined anechoic SOL with posterior acoustic enhancement seen in upper pole of right kidney

Medullary Cysts

a. Medullary sponge kidney.
b. Cysts associated with uremia/dialysis.
c. Pyelogenic cysts.
d. Papillary necrosis.

Miscellaneous

a. Inflammatory (TB, hydatid).
b. Neoplastic (Renal cell carcinoma, Wilm's tumor, multilocular cystic nephroma).
c. Trauma (resolved hematoma).

Extrarenal Cysts

a. Peripelvic.
b. Parapelvic.
c. Perinephric.

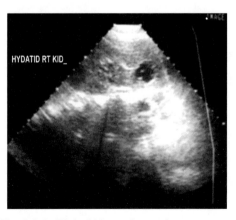

Fig. 8.2.2: Right kidney shows the presence of hydatid cyst with 3 daughter cysts inside it

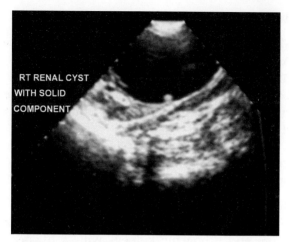

Fig. 8.2.3: A large anechoic cyst is seen occupying the lower and middle pole of right kidney with a mural nodule inside it—renal cell carcinoma

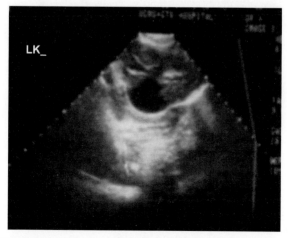

Fig. 8.2.4: Urinoma—a small anechoic collection is seen to communicate with pelvicalyceal system of right kidney

Multicystic Dysplastic Kidney

- Most common cystic disease in infant and fetus
- Associated with oligohydramnios
- 20 percent bilateral
- Lobulated kidney having multiple small to large cysts separated by strands of abnormal parenchymal.

Infantile Autosomal Recessive Polycystic Kidney Disease

- Bilateral, symmetrical
- Tiny radial cysts due to dilated collecting tubules
- Large and echogenic kidneys with a hypoechoic rim
- In mild disease only the medulla is affected.

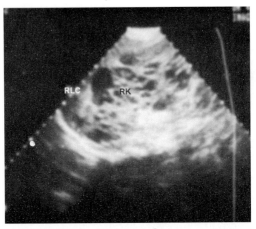

Fig. 8.2.5: Adult polycystic kidney disease—a classical case of APKD showing innumerable cyst with complete architectural distortion of the right kidney. The kidney is also enlarged

Adult Autosomal Dominant Polycystic Kidney Disease

- Occurs due to a defect in formation of basement membrane collagen
- Multiple, bilateraly, asymmetrical cysts of different sizes are seen
- Kidney size is increased
- Both cortex and medulla are affected
- Normal renal parenchyma is seen.

Rauines Modification of Bear's Criteria for Diagnosis of ADPCKD

Age	Family history	Number of cyst	Kidney affected
< 30 yr	+	>2	U/L or B/L
31-59 yr	+	> 2 + 2	B/L
>60 yr	+	> 4 + 4	B/L

Medullary Sponge Kidney

- Occur due to ectesia and elongation of medullary tubules.
- Dystrophic calcification in walls.
- Rarely cysts are seen separately only echogenic kidney are seen.

Uremia Associated Cystic Disease

- Occurs due to ischemia associated with dialysis
- Cyst may occur both in cortex and medulla and increase in size with time

- Association of adenoma and renal cell carcinoma are well known.

8.3 DIFFERENTIAL DIAGNOSIS OF COMPLEX/SOLID RENAL MASSES

Benign

1. Oncocytoma and adenoma.
2. Angiomyolipoma.
3. Reninoma.
4. Mesoblastic nephroma.
5. Multilocular cystic nephroma.
6. Hemangioma, aneurysm, AVM, hematoma.

Malignant

1. Wilm's tumor.
2. Renal cell carcinoma.
3. Squamous cell carcinoma.
4. Soft tissue sarcomas.
5. Lymphoma.
6. Leukemia.
7. Metastasis.
8. Transitional cell carcinoma.

Oncocytoma/Adenoma

- Oncocytoma is an eosinophilic adenoma, both are usually benign tumors arising from proximal convoluted tubules
- Sharply defined masses of variable echogenicity and peripheral spoke wheel pattern of blood vessels.

Mesoblastic Nephroma

- Commonest solid tumor in first month of life hence known as congenital Wilms' tumor
- Appearance is similar to Wilm's and differentiation on USG is not possible
- Calcification is rare.

Multilocular Cystic Nephroma

- Known as cystic Wilms' tumor and benign cystic nephroma
- May have calcification in wall and indent the pelvicalyceal system causing obstruction.

Angiomyolipoma

- Females, solitary
- 20 percent associated with tuberous sclerosis
- Localy invasive
- Fat is a very specific feature.

Transitional Cell Carcinoma

- Punctate coarse calcification
- Hypovascular
- Intrapelvic/intracalyceal mass invading the parenchyma.
- May form a terminal dilated calyx known as onco-calyx.

Wilms' Tumor

- Most common intrarenal malignancy of childhood.

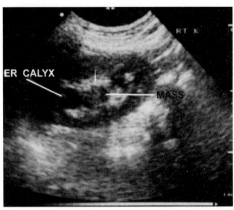

Fig. 8.3.1: Transitional cell carcinoma—a hypoechoic mass is seen spliting the central sinus echocomplex and causing focal caliectasis of the upper pole of right kidney

- 5-10 percent are bilateral, 5-10 percent have calcification.
- Echogenic mass, well defined with a halo of compressed tissue around it.
- Sonolucent lakes of large size are common.

Renal Cell Carcinoma

- Most common (86%) of all renal tumors
- Arising from tubular epithelium
- Peak age = 50-70 years
- Males three times more
- Basically an echogenic lesion with hypoechoic rim
- Areas of necrosis may be seen
- 3-7 percent lesion are near totaly cystic.
  — All the malignant lesions have a non specific appearance of a hypoechoic space occupying lesion.

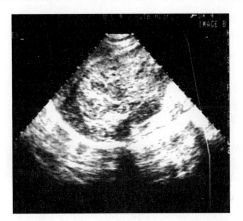

Fig. 8.3.2: A heterogenous echotexture SOL is seen in the region of upper middle pole of right kidney

8.4 DIFFERENTIAL DIAGNOSIS OF HYPOECHOIC RENAL SINUS

1. All causes of pelvicaliectasis

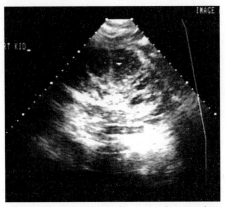

Fig. 8.4.1: Pyonephrosis-stone is seen in renal pelvis with pelvicalyceal hydronephrosis with evidence of debris and air inside it

2. Transitional cell carcinoma.
3. Pyonephrosis.
4. Prominent vessels in sinus.
5. Parapelvic peripelvic cyst.
6. Blood clot at pelvis.
   — Description of these condition are given in respective sections.

8.5 DIFFERENTIAL DIAGNOSIS OF HYPERECHOIC RENAL NODULES

1. Complicated cystic lesion:
   • When there is hemorrhage within a cyst.
2. Inflammatory masses in kidney formed in cases of tuberculosis, malakoplakia, xanthogranulomatous pyelonephritis, fungal infection, schistosomiasis.
3. AIDS related conditions like nephrocalcinosis, acute tubular necrosis, interstitial nephritis, *Candida*, CMV, *Cryptococcus*, *Pneumocystis*, MAIC, lymphoma, Kaposi's sarcoma.
4. Gas loculi seen in cases of emphysematous pyelonephritis.
5. Calcified tumoral components in Wilms' tumor, RCC, TCC, etc.
6. Calcified vascular lesions like AVM, aneurysm.
7. Fat containing tumors like Wilm's tumor, oncocytoma and angiomyolipoma.
8. Parenchymal calcification in TB, schistosomiasis, nephrocalcinosis.
9. Metastatic deposits may sometimes be hyperechoic.
10. Small RCC.

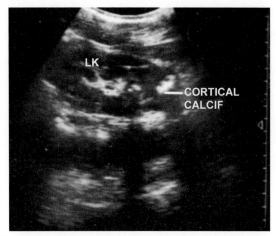

Fig. 8.5.1: Renal calculus: Dense echogenic focus with distal acoustic shadowing is seen in the renal cortex suggestive of old tubercular involvement. A calculus is also seen in lower pole

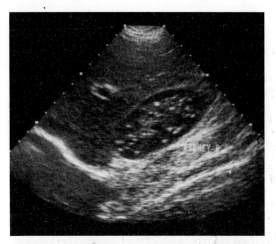

Fig. 8.5.2: Nephrocalcinosis-stippled calcification is seen in the region of the renal pyramid

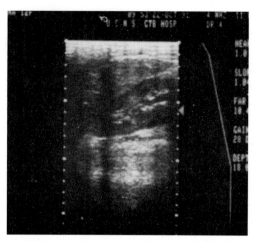

Fig. 8.5.3A: A mild hydronephrosis—minimal splitting of the pelvicalyceal system is noted

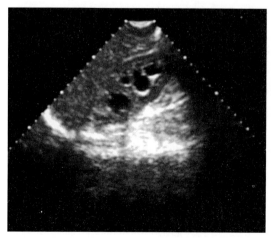

Fig. 8.5.3B: Moderate hydronephrosis

8.6 DIFFERENTIAL DIAGNOSIS OF DILATED PELVICALYCEAL SYSTEM AND URETER

1. Stricture at infundibulum, pelviureteric junction, ureter, this could be due to tumor, calculus or infection.
2. Extrinsic vascular compression occurs most commonly at right upper pole calyx known as Fraley syndrome.

    Similar compression on ureter may occur due to retrocaval ureter or even a large aortic aneurysm.
3. Hydrocalycosis megacalyx, boggy pelvis and megaureter are congenital conditions leading to isolated dilatation of the involved parts. Megacalyx = >12 upto 20-25.

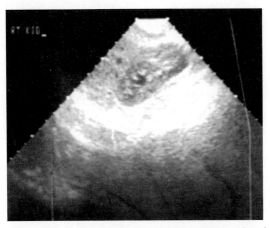

Fig. 8.6.1: Focal caliectasis seen in upper pole of right kidney, old case of TB kidney

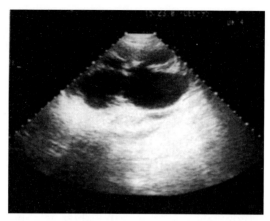

Fig. 8.6.2: PUJ obstruction—longitudinal scan showing gross pelvic dilatation and dilated calyces due to pelviureteric obstruction

4. Retroperitoneal fibrosis
   • Leads to medial deviation and partial obstruction of ureter at L4/5 level.
5. Calculus disease—all calculi whether radio-opaque or not are seen as hyperechoic structures.
6. Post-obstructive atrophy due to volume lose and negative force leads to dilated PCS or calyx.
7. Blood clot in the lumen.
8. Sloughed papilla in the lumen.
9. Edema of walls.
10. Trauma.
11. Retroperitoneal masses.
12. Transitional cell carcinoma.
13. Vescicoureteric reflux.
14. Postpartum upto 6 months.
15. Following urinary tract infection.

9

Urinary Bladder

9.1 DIFFERENTIAL DIAGNOSIS OF BLADDER WALL THICKENING

Diffuse Thickening: > 3 mm

1. Acute cystitis.
2. Schistosomiasis.
3. Tuberculosis.
4. Radiation cystitis.
5. Cyclophosphamide cystitis.
6. Malakoplakia.

Focal Thickening/Masses

1. Nephrogenic adenoma.
2. Transitional cell papilloma.
3. Transitional cell carcinoma.
4. Squamous cell carcinoma.
5. Adenocarcinoma.
6. Leiomyoma/Leiomyosarcoma.
7. Rhabdomyosarcoma.
8. Hemangioma.
9. Paraganglioma.
10. Invasion by pelvic malignancies.

11. Secondary deposits:
    - Systemic
    - Lymphoma.
12. Cystitis glandularis and cystitis cystica.
13. Schistosomiasis.
14. Spread of extravesicle inflammation from diverticulitis, Crohn's disease, appendicitis, urachal abscess, pelvic inflammatory disease.
15. Endometriosis.
16. Chronic cystitis: May represent as focal thickening or solid projecting masses and difficult to differentiate from malignancy.
17. Adherent clot.

Acute Cystitis

- Transurethral extension of infection.

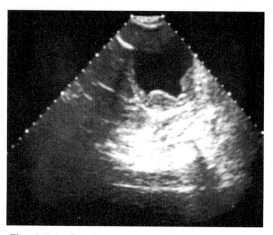

Fig. 9.1.1: Carcinoma—irregular wall thickening seen on posterior wall

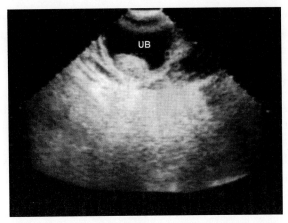

Fig. 9.1.2: Clot in urinary bladder is seen as a large echogenic lesion in relation to the posterior wall of urinary bladder

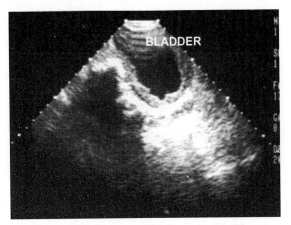

Fig. 9.1.3: Cystitis—the wall of urinary bladder are irregularly thickened

- Females more than males
- Most commonly *E.coli*

- Gas in the lumen and in the wall is seen in emphysematous cystitis. This occurs in immunocompromised patients.

Schistosomiasis

- A disease of submucosa and lamina propria leading to mucosal ulcerations and malignancies in late phases
- Diffuse, irregular wall thickening associated with lumpy, sometimes polypoidal granulomas and straky curvilinear calcification is the hallmark
- Eventually the bladder becomes small and fibrotic.

Tuberculosis

- A process that descends from upper tract and so the earliest changes are seen at ureteral orifices whereby they spread centrifugally
- Diffuse but lumpy thickening with calcification in late stages is seen
- Small fibrosed bladder is the terminal event.

Cyclophosphamide Cystitis

- Acute—edematous, hyperemic, ulcerated mucosa with intraluminal clots
- Chronic—small fibrose bladder.
  - Malignancy.

Malakoplakia

- An uncommon granulomatous respone to UTI especially to that caused by *E.coli*

- Females; 5th-6th decades
- Associated with diabetes, alchoholism, liver disease, mycobacterial infection, sarcoidosis and post-transplant
- 5-3 cm, solitary/multiple mural based masses with mural thickening.

Radiation Cystitis

- Acute—like any other diffuse cystitis
- Chronic—occurs on an average after four years
- No specific feature is seen.

Cystitis Cystica and Cystitis Glandularis

- Occur due to chronic cystitis causing cystic change and later on glandular change in Brunn's nest (urothelial cell rest in submucosa)
- Difficult to differentiate from malignancy and may lead to adenocarcinoma
- Cyst (intramural) and solid papillary masses with wall thickening may be seen.

Endometriosis

- Most common site for endometriotic deposits in urinary tract is bladder
- Serosal deposits protruding into lumen or even intraluminal deposits may be seen.

Paraganglioma

- Trigone is the most common location followed by dome and lateral walls
- Lesion is vascular.

Hemangioma

- Dome and posterolateral walls
- Two types of appearance:
  1. A rounded, well defined, hyperechoic solid mass in lumen showing in vascularity in Doppler.
  2. Diffuse wall thickening with hypoechoic spaces and calcification.

Adenocarcinoma

- Has to be differentiated from adenocarcinoma elsewhere infiltrating.
- Associated stone/calcification is a feature.

Squamous Cell Carcinoma

- Large, solid, infiltrative lesion.

Transitional Cell Carcinoma

- Men, 6th-7th decades, trigone/posterolateral walls
- 70 percent superficial, rest are invasive
- USG is 95 percent sensitive in its detection.
- Presents as a focal non-mobile mass/wall thickening.

9.2 DIFFERENTIAL DIAGNOSIS OF BLADDER CONTOUR AND CALIBER ABNORMALITY

Symmetric Narrowing

1. Pelvic lipomatosis.
2. Pelvic hematoma.

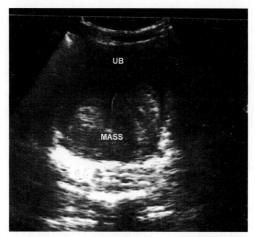

Fig. 9.1.4: Transitional cell carcinoma—a polypoidal mass is seen to arise from post wall of urinary bladder

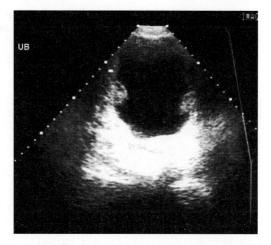

Fig. 9.1.5: Multifocal carcinoma—transverse scan of UB showing nodular growth at two different regions

3. Lymphoma.
4. Iliopsoas hypertrophy.
5. Narrow bony pelvis.
6. Nonlymphomatous lymphadenopathy.
7. Lymphocele/lymphangioma.
8. Iliac artery aneurysm.
9. Iliac vein varices.
10. Seminal vescicle cysts.

Asymmetric Narrowing/Contour

1. Diverticulum.
2. Fistula.
3. Hernia.
   — In all above conditions the dome is tapering while the base is rounded due to external compression.

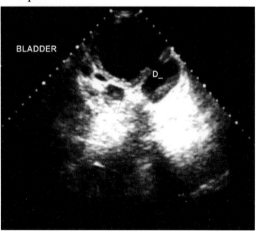

Fig. 9.2.1: Narrow neck diverticulum as seen from the posterior wall of urinary bladder with evidence of debris inside

— Mucosa is uniformly normal.

Pelvic Lipomatosis

- Black, males
- Proliferation of fat in pelvica seen as echogenic tissue compressing the bladder symmetrically.
- A pear shapped/tear drop bladder ureter and elongated recto-sigmoid.

Pelvic Hematoma

- History of blunt abdominal trauma is important.
- Less echogenicity of extravescile tissue is the only factor that differentiates it.

Lymphoma

- Involving pelvic nodes causes symmetric narrowing.

Iliopsoas Hypertrophy

- Young athletic individual
- The deviation of mid ureter clinches the diagnosis.

Adrenal

10.1 BILATERAL LARGE ADRENAL

- Lymphoma
- Hyperplasia
- Hemorrhage

Infections

- Tuberculosis
- Histoplasmosis
- Immunodeficiency states.
- Pheochromocytoma (10%)
- Adenomas (10%)
- Metastasis
- Wolman's disease

Lymphoma

Non-Hodgkin's is the most common cell type.

On sonography they appear as bilateral enlarged adrenal with discrete or conglomerate hypoechoic masses. Masses may be so hypoechoic as to stimulate cysts. The medulla cannot be differentiated from the cortex as in any other infiltration process.

Hyperplasia

Congenital adrenal hyperplasia is an autosomal recessive condition clinically presenting with features of visualization or salt loss depending upon the hormone which is deficit. Both adrenals are enlarged but the differentiation of medulla and cortex is preserved.

Hemorrhage Adrenal hemorrhage may be spontaneous or post-traumatic. Sonographic appearance of acute hemorrhage is a bright echogenic mass in the adrenal bed, which becomes smaller and anechoic with time. Patients with B/L hemorrhage are at increased risk for development of acute adrenal insufficiency.

Infections Tuberculosis-may cause bilateral diffuse, inhomogenous enlargement of adrenals. Punctate calcification may also be seen. Infection of adrenal glands are seen in association with AIDS and organ transplantation. Common offending organisms are fungi, mycobacteria, CMV, herpes, toxiplasmosis, etc. On ultrasound bilateral adrenal glands shows heterogeneously Hypoechoic masses. On formation of abscesses gas may be demonstrated in the lesion.

Pheochromocytoma

They are usually solitary but in 10 percent cases they are bilateral.

Sonographically most are large and well margi-nated. Either homogenous or heterogeneous (b/o necrosis and hemorrhage) solid masses.

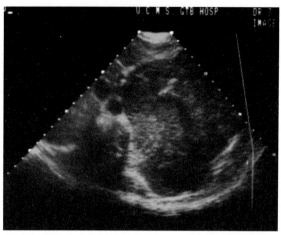

Fig. 10.1.1: A large predominantly hypoechoic well defined left adrenal mass lesion seen with evidence of calcification in it

Metastasis

The most common primary tumors to give rise to adrenal metastasis are lung, breast, melanoma, kidney, thyroid and colon cancers.

May be unilateral or bilateral.

On ultrasound appears as solid masses round to oval hypoechoic lesions. They may show inhomogeniety due to necrosis and hemorrhage.

Wolman's Disease

This is a rare autosomal recessive lipid storage disease. Infants less than 6 months of age show marked hepatosplenomegaly and massive B/L adrenal gland enlargement.

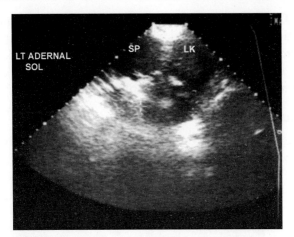

Fig. 10.1.2: Metastases—a hypoechoic mass with irregular outline is seen in the region of left adrenal in a case of bronchogenic carcinoma

10.2 UNILATERAL ADRENAL MASSES

- Pheochromocytoma
- Lymphoma
- Adenoma
- Neuroblastoma
- Myelolipoma
- Hemorrhage
- Adrenocarcinoma
- Metastasis

Adenoma

Adrenal adenoma may be hyperfunctioning or non-hyperfunctioning. Hyperfunctioning adenomas give rise to Cushing's syndrome or Conn's disease.

On sonography they appear as solid, small, round and well defined lesions. Right upper quadrant retroperitoneal fat reflection is displaced posteriorly by hepatic or subhepatic masses while kidney and adrenal masses displace it anteriorly.

Neuroblastoma

The second most common abdominal tumor of child-hood. Thirty percent occurring in childrens < 5 yr. On

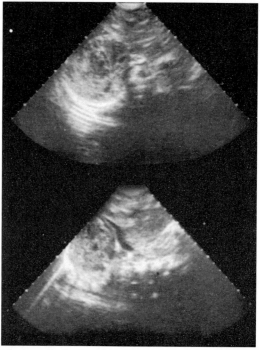

Fig. 10.2.1: Longitudinal and transverse scan of abdomen of a 6-month old child with marked heterogenicity and areas of high reflectivity within it—neuroblastoma

ultrasound, they are seen as on poorly defined and heterogenous lesion with areas of calcification, hemorrhage and necrosis. The lesion often crosses the midline and causes displacement and compression of ipsilateral kidney without otherwise distorting the internal renal architecture. They also tends to spread early and widely—spreads around aorta, celiac, SMA arteries.

Pheochromocytoma are hyperfunctioning tumor-secreting norepinephrine and epinephrine and showing features of episodic hypertension, palpitation with tachycardia, headache. Sonography demonstrate large, well marginated heterogenous (due to necrosis and hemorrhage) solid lesions. Ten percent lesions may demonstrate calcification.

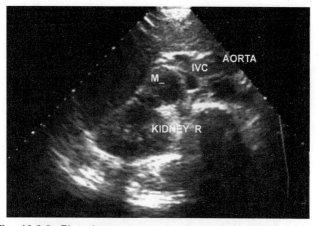

Fig. 10.2.2: Pheochromocytoma—a hypoechoic rounded well-defined lesion with uniform echogenicity is seen in the right adrenal gland

Myelolipoma

Adrenal myelolipomas are rare benign nonhyperfunctioning tumors composed of fat and bone marrow elements.

On sonography an echogenic mass with apparent diaphragmatic discursion is diagnostic of the condition. Tumor may appear isoechoic if composed predominantly of myeloid element.

Adrenocarcinoma rare malignant tumors. It may arise from any of the layers of adrenal cortex.

Hyperfunctioning tumors are small and homogeneous in echo pattern, similar to renal cortex.

The nonhyperfunctioning tumors are larger and heterogeneous with central areas of necrosis and hemorrhage. All lesions tend to be well defined with a

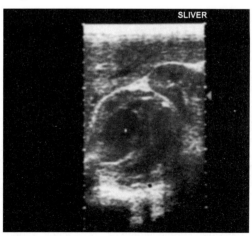

Fig. 10.2.3: A solid heterogenous mass with a well defined echogenic capsule and cystic areas of necrosis

lobulated border. Calcification may be seen in 20 percent cases. A surrounding thin echogenic vascular capsule is a specific feature of adrenal cortical carcinoma.

10.3 LARGE SOLID ADRENAL MASSES

- Cortical carcinoma.
- Pheochromocytoma.
- Neuroblastoma.
- Ganglioneuroma.
- Myelolipoma.
- Metastasis.
- Hemangiomas—may become large in size. They have nonspecific US features with cystic, solid or complex appearances. Phleboliths may be seen within the lesions—inlammation/infection—tuberculosis, abscess.

Ganglioneuroma is a rare benign adrenal neoplasm. It is slow growing and clinically silent until pressure symptoms are evident. Sonographically they appear homogenously solid and change shape rather than displacing adjacent organs.

10.4 CYSTIC ADRENAL MASSES

Adrenal Cyst

- Rare benign lesion, found incidently
- Typically unilateral but bilateral in 15 percent of cases

- Most common in 3rd to 4th decades and show a female preponderance.

Sonographically they are round or oval with a thin smooth wall. Good through-transmission is present but often internal debris is noted.

According to their origin they are classified as:

1. Endothelial—most common variety and include angiomatous, lymphangiectatic and hamartomatous lesions.
2. Pseudocysts—secondary to hemorrhage into a normal adrenal gland, i.e old hemorrhage or tumor-cystic adenoma-neuroblastoma.
3. Epithelial cysts
4. Parasitic—echinococcal cyst.

10.5 ADRENAL PSUEDOMASSES

Structures that may simulate adrenal masses include:
- Thickened diaphragmatic crura
- Accessory spleen
- Gastric fundus
- Gastric diverticulum
- Renal vein
- Retrocrural and retroperitoneal lymphadenopathy
- Upper pole renal cysts and renal tumors
- Pancreatic tumors
- Hypertrophied caudate lobe of liver
- Fluid filled colon interposed between stomach and kidney.

11

Peritoneal and Mesenteric Masses

11.1 ROUND SOLID MASSES IN MESENTERY

— Metastasis
— Lymphoma
— Leiomyosarcoma
- Metastasis from colon and ovary. Metastasis due to intraperitoneal seedlings are seen in primary mucinous tumors of ovary, appendix, colon and breast
- Lymphoma: Lymphoma may present as a endo-exoenteric mass with a solid mass in the mesentery and adjacent small bowel mass
- Leiomyosarcoma: Of small bowel is most commonly seen in ileum. The large extrinsic component of the lesion is seen as a well-defined solid mesenteric mass with areas of necrosis
- Neural tumors
- Lipoma
- Fibrous histiocytoma
- Hemangioma
- Desmoid tumors

- Mesenteritis: Various conditions like Crohn's, trauma, surgery and pancreatitis may cause inflammation and thickening of the mesentery which on US may appear as a focal echopoor mass. This may also be seen as a part of retroperitoneal fibrosis.

11.2 ILL DEFINED MASS

- Metastasis
  - Direct extension from adjacent neoplasm (ovary uterus, pancreas) may infiltrate the mesentery.

Lymphoma Infilterating small bowel lymphoma is plaque like involvement of the bowel wall and may be associated with desmoplastic reaction involving the mesentery.

The mesenteric lymph node involvement may be seen as an ill-defined component mass engulfing and encasing adjacent normal loops.

Carcinoid

- Lymphoma—Infiltrating small bowel lymphoma is plaque like involvement of the bowel wall and may be associated with dismoplastic reaction involving the mesentery. The mesenteric lymph node involvement may be seen in ill defined confluent mass engulfing and encasing adjacent bowel loops.
- Fibromatosis
- Chronic or retractile mesenteritis, fibrosing mesenteritis: Retractile mesenteritis also called as chronic

fibrosing mesenteritis or mesenteric hypodystrophy is a rare condition of unknown etiology causing fibrofatty thickening of the small bowel mesentery. On ultrasound it may be seen as a nonspecific illdefined (hypoechoic or heterogenous) lesion at the root of the mesentery extending till the bowel border

- Lipodystrophy
- Peritoneal mesothelioma
- Fibrotic reaction of carcinoid
- Desmoid tumors.

Liposarcoma

Diffuse infiltrative lipomatosis.
- Tuberculosis
- Diverticulitis
- Pancreatitis.

11.3 LOCULATED CYSTIC PERITONEAL MASSES

- i. Mesenteric: Lymphangioma, mesenteric cyst, mesenteric hematoma.
- ii. Pseudomyxoma peritonei.
- iii. Intra-abdominal abscess.
- iv. Lymphocele.
- v. Meconium peritonitis.
- vi. Peritoneal tuberculosis.
- vii. Omental cyst.
- viii. Cystic mesothelioma.
- ix. Cystic spindle shaped tumors.

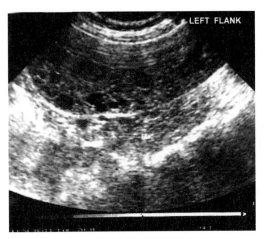

Fig. 11.3.1: Intraperitoneal hydatid—extends from the spleen to pelvis occupying whole of left flank. The lower pole of mass showed an rounded lesion with multiple daughter cyst in it

    x. Paracardiac pseudocyst
   xi. Intraperitoneal hydatid.

11.4 SOLID PERITONEAL LESIONS

    i. Mesothelioma.
   ii. Carcinomatosis.
  iii. Pseudomyxoma peritonei.
  iv. Leiomyomatosis peritoneal disseminata.

Mesenteric Cyst

- Usually found in the root of the mesentery
- Sonographically it appears as unilocular cystic lesion.

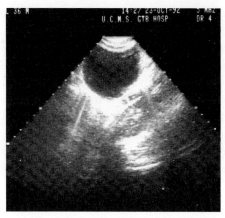

Fig. 11.4.1: Mesenteric cyst—a large cystic anechoic SOL with thin wall seen displacing the bowel loops

That may be septated, rarely a fat fluid level may be seen. When differentiation from solid peritoneal lesions and mesenteric cystic teratoma becomes difficult.

1. Desmoid tumors.
2. Occurs most commonly in abdominal wall.
3. Occurs in mesentery also.
4. Mesenteric dermoids are hypoechoic masses with area of messenteric shadowing due to fibrous tissue.

Mesenteric lymphangioma are multiseptated lesions, which can attain large size and change shape. They have minimal noneffect on the adjacent bowel and no displacement of the mesenteric vessels is seen.

Intraperitoneal Abscess

These develop usually following surgery, bowel perforation trauma, pancreatitis or in patients with decreased immune response. The majority develop in the upper and down and on right side.

A loculated fluid collection containing gas bubbles (echogenic foci with reverbelization artefacts) is strongly systemic of an abscess. Ultrasound may reveal this typical appearance or it may be seen as on ovoid or irregularly shaped collection with debris, debris-fluid level or septations. A complex appearance with solid and cystic components can also be seen. Some abscess may simulate on echogenic solid mass.

Lymphocele

Surgery or trauma cause disruption of lymphatic vessels resulting in lymph-collection. They are most commonly seen in pelvis or intraperitoneal recesses.

They usually appear as anechoic collection or variable size. Large collections can cause significant pressure symptoms complicated lymphocele contains debris or septae.

Meconium Peritonitis

Antenatal bowel perforation spill meconium into the peritoneal cavity which incites a foreign body reaction resulting in formation of a cystic or complex mass having echogenic walls.

Intestinal stenosis/atresia and meconium ileus are the common causes.

Occurs most commonly in the abdominal wall, but also in the mesentery. Mesenteric dermoid tumors are hypoechoic masses with areas of acoustic shadowing due to fibrotic tissue.

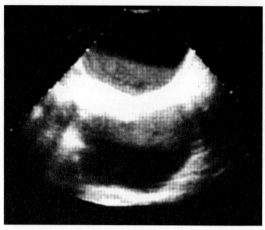

Fig. 11.4.2: Pelvic abscess-fluid debris level is seen inside it

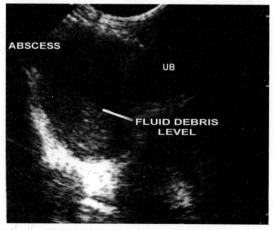

Fig. 11.4.3: Debris-fluid level seen inside a collection in the pelvis

Lymphoma

- Most common primary mesenteric malignancy
- Isolated enlarged lymph nodes measuring more than 1.5 cm in diameter are seen around the celiac axis
- SMA, and in porta hepatic
- They are often hypoechoic
- Lobulated mass encasing the mesenteric vessels that manifests as linear echoes within the mass-referred to as 'sandwich sign'
- May present as a exophytic mass in bowel wall with a solid mass in the mesentery.

Mesothelioma

- Is a sarcoma arising from the serous membrane.
- Closely related to asbestos exposure
- Thickening of the omentum forming a omental mantle or cake is evident on US. This appearance is also seen in tuberculosis or peritoneal carcinomatous.
- Minimal ascites
- Liver metastasis
- Pleural plaques and effusion small nodules may be identified on peritoneal surface or in mesenteric fat.

Cystic Mesothelioma

Very rare neoplasm of the peritoneum. It has no association with asbestos exposure.

Peritoneal tuberculosis may be caused by direct spread of bowel tuberculosis or by hematogenous dissemination of a lung lesion. On sonography a loculated fluid collecion with septae and debris may be seen. Associated features are mesenteric lymph-

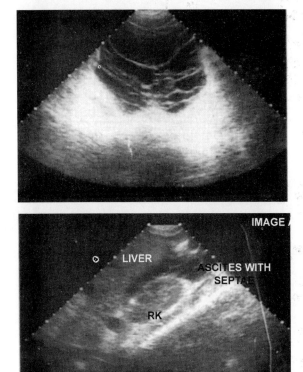

Fig. 11.4.4: Ascites with multiple thick internal septae seen in (A) pelvis and (B) hepatorenal pouch

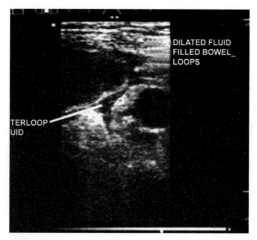

Fig. 11.4.5A: Abdominal tuberculosis: Interloop
fluid between loops

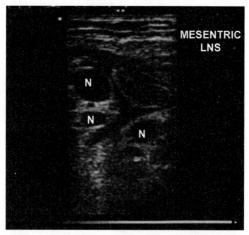

Fig. 11.4.5B: Abdominal tuberculosis: Multiple hypoechoic well-
defined lesion seen in the mesentery suggestive of lymph nodes

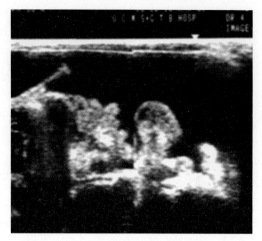

Fig. 11.4.6: Ascites outlining bowel loops

adenopathy, omental case, bowel thickening and ascites.

Omental Cyst

On ultrasound this appears as a well defined, rounded, anechoic lesion present close to the bowel wall. This resembles a mesenteric cyst which is present in the root of the mesentery.

Pancreatic Pseudocyst

Pancreatic pseudocysts are collection of pancreatic fluid with a high amylase content surrounded by a fibrosis wall. These develop in 50 percent of patients 2 to 3 weeks after an attack of acute pancreatitis. On US they appear as a well defined, walled off anechoic collection

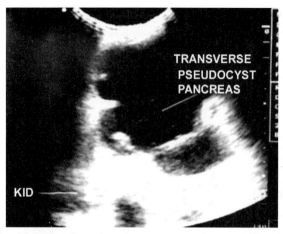

Fig. 11.4.7A: Pseudocyst pancreas—a large multiloculated collection seen in lesser sac with evidence of debris in it

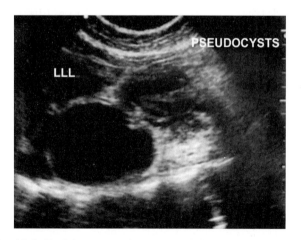

Fig. 11.4.7B: A large pseudocyst seen in lesser sac posterior to left lobe of liver. Another pseudocyst is seen adjacent to it with evidence of internal septae

most commonly seen in the lesser sac. Few dependent debris may be evident. Septae and echoes develop within it following infection. Other features or complications of pancreatitis may also be evident.

Metastasis

Metastasis to the peritoneum and mesentery usually arises due to intraperitoneal readings from a variety of sources most common being carcinoma of ovary and GIT and breast.

On U/S thickened sheet like greater omentum (secondary to infiltration by metastasis cells) appear as "omental mangle or cake". In the presence of ascites small nodules attached to the peritoneal surface are seen clearly.

Enlarged isolated mesenteric lymph nodes or conglomerated hypoechoic lymph node may be evident masses.

Psuedomyxoma Peritonei

Characterized by mucinous peritoneal implants and gelatinous ascites.

Most often caused by secondary metastasis from mucin producing adenocarcinoma of ovary, appendix, colon and rectum. Hypoechoic to strongly echogenic nodular masses distributed throughout the peritoneal cavity. These deposits characteristically scalloping the adjacent liver surface.

Leiomyomatosis peritonealis disseminated: This condition occurs in pregnant or women of child bearing age group. Disseminated solid benign leiomyoma are seen a solid peritoneal masses. Ascites is usually not present.

Diffuse infilterative lipomatosis This rare disease entity affects young people is characterized by overgrowth of fat in the retroperitoneum. On US an echogenic mass is evident which cannot be differentiated from liposarcoma.

12.1 DIFFERENTIAL DIAGNOSIS OF ACUTE SCROTUM

Causes

1. Testicular torsion.
2. Epididymitis with or without orchitis.
3. Torsion of testicular appendages.
4. Testicular trauma.
5. Acute hydrocele.
6. Incarcerated hernia.
7. Idiopathic scrotal edema.
8. Henöch-Schonlein purpura.
9. Scrotal fat necrosis.
10. Familial mediterranean fever.
11. Abdominal pathology.

Testicular Torsion

- Normal size and appearance early
- Hypoechoic after 4-6 hr due to edema
- Heterogenous after 24 hours due to hemorrhage and infarction known as missed torsion
- Hypoechoic epididymis

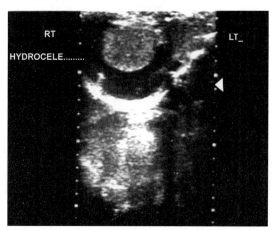

Fig. 12.1.1: Transverse section of right scrotal sac showing hydrocele

- Reactive hydrocele
- Skin thickening
- Enlarged twisted spermatic cord.

Epididymitis with or without Orchitis

- The part affected is bulky, heterogenous and hypoechoic
- Associated reactive hydrocele, skin-thickening
- Increased/normal color flow is the point of differentiation from torsion.
- Infarction and abscess are the complications.

Torsion of Testicular Appendage

- Variable sized, ovoid to round, mobile hypoechoic mass with hyperechoic rim.

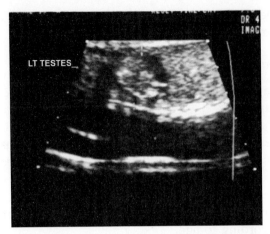

Fig. 12.1.2A: Epididymis is swollen with a collection adjacent to it with internal echoes—epididymitis with scrotal abscess

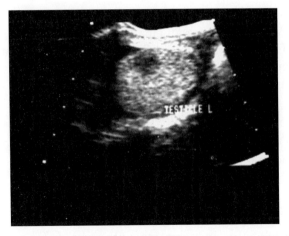

Fig. 12.1.2B: Epididymis is swollen and shows a hypoechoic lesion in. Testis also shows hypoechoic lesion. FNAC confirmed tubercular epididymo-orchitis

- Decreased internal and increased external vascularity.

Testicular Trauma

- Pathologies that occur are hematoma, fracture, rupture
- A ruptured testes is ill defined, hypoechoic, heterogenous with loss of normal contour and ruptured tunica. Seminiferous tubules may be extruded
- Fracture may or may not be seen as a hypoechoic line
- Hematoma is seen as a mass of variable appearance according to age.

Idiopathic Scrotal Edema

- Between 5-11 year age
- Pain, swelling, erythema
- Thickened scrotal wall with normal testes and epididymis
- Increase/normal color flow in wall.

Henöch-Schonlein Purpura

- Diffusely swollen scrotum and its contents with normal color flow/increased flow
- Resolves completely and spontaneously.

Abdominal Pathology

- Especially in neonates with patent processus vaginalis.

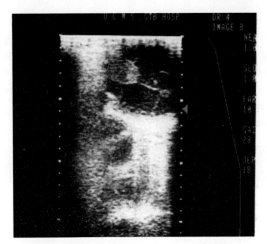

Fig. 12.1.3A: Organized scrotal hematoma

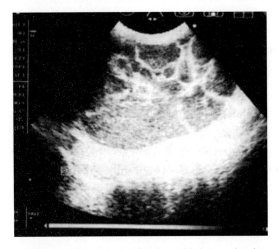

Fig. 12.1.3B: Multiloculated collection with internal echoes seen in the left scrotal sac pushing the testis to one corner—organized hematoma

- Conditions that can cause secondary symptoms in scrotum are adrenal hemorrhage, delayed spleen rupture of battered baby, hepatic laceration, Crohn's disease, acute appendicitis, appendix perforation
- Scrotal vein thrombosis due to catheterization of femoral vein during cardiac catheterization is an unusual cause.

12.2 DIFFERENTIAL DIAGNOSIS OF SCROTAL CALCIFICATION

Testicular Calcifications

- Infective: Granuloma, tuberculosis, filariasis, sarcoidosis
- Vascular: Infarcts, vascular malformation arterial wall
- Testicular microlithiasis
- Neoplasms: Burnt out germ cell tumor, large Sertoli cell tumors, teratoma/teratocarcinoma gonadoblastoma.

Extratesticular Calcifications

- Chronic epididymitis
- Scrotal pearls
- Schistosomiasis
- Hematomas
- Meconium peritonitis.

Testicular Microlithiasis

- Calcified specks within seminiferous tubules.
- Corpora-amylacea-like bodies formed.

- Associated with cryptorchidism, Kleinfelter's syndrome, tumors, pseudohermaphroditism
- Echogenic specks with comet tail artefact and no shadow.
- Bilateral.
- Follow-up 6 monthly with tumor marker evaluation is a must.

Isolated Microlithiasis

- Fewer than fine simple calcification.

Scrotal Pearls

- Parts of tunica break loose when inflamed or even from a tarted appendix testes/epididymis
- Lie between two layers of tunica with associated hydrocele
- Consists of hydroxyapetite core with fibrinoid material deposited around it.

Sarcoidosis

- Epididymal involvement more than testicular
- Recurrant painless inflammation, enlargement.

12.3 DIFFERENTIAL DIAGNOSIS OF SCROTAL GAS

1. Infection by gas forming bacteria:
   — Associated calcification, fluid, thickened wall/tunica.
   — Testes is bulky and hypoechoic.

— Heterogenous echotexture.
— Flow increased.

2. Hernia of bowel loops if processus vaginalis is patent:
   — Intrascrotal peristalsis is confirmatory.
3. Trauma/intervention.
4. Pneumoperitoneum with patent PV.

12.4 DIFFERENTIAL DIAGNOSIS OF SCROTAL MASSES

INTRATESTICULAR

a. Secondary: Metastasis, lymphoma, leukemia.
b. Primary:
   — Malignant

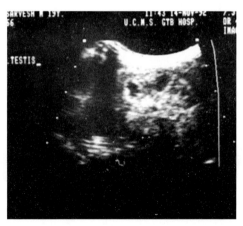

Fig. 12.4.1: Testicular malignacy—right testis is replaced by a solid mass of heterogeneous echotexture with few hypoechoic, anecholic and hyperechoic areas

Germ Cell Tumors

90-95 percent mostly malignant.

    i. Tumors of one histologic type:

- Seminoma
  — classical
  — spermatocytic.
- Embryonal cell carcinoma—adult type
  — infantile type
  — endodermal sinus tumor (yolk sac tumor)
- Teratoma—mature
  — immature
  — with malignant transformation.
  — choriocarcinoma.

    ii. Tumors of more than one histologic type:

- Teratocarcinoma (teratoma with embryonal cell carcinoma).
- Any other combination.

Gonadal Stromal Tumor

- 3-6 percent, mostly benign
- Leydig cell tumor
- Sertoli's cell tumor
- Granulosa cell tumor
- Theca cell tumor
- Tumors of primitive gonadal stroma
- Mixed.

BENIGN

- Simple cyst
- Epidermoid cyst

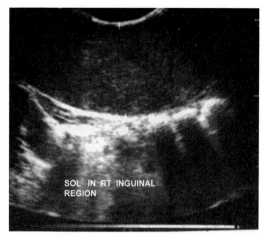

Fig. 12.4.2A(i): Well-defined round homogenous echotexture SOL seen in the right inguinal region

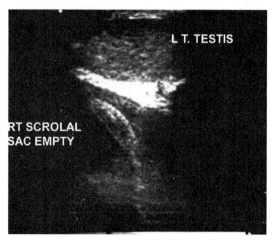

Fig. 12.4.2A(ii): The right scrotal sac is empty and left testis is normal in position

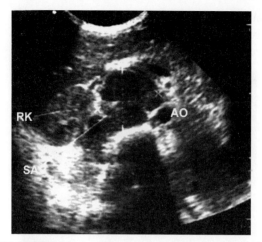

Fig. 12.4.2A(iii): There are para-aortic lymph nodes. Excision biopsy from the lesion revealed seminoma testis

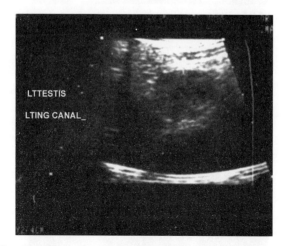

Fig. 12.4.2B: Left ectopic testis lying in the inguinal canal

- Cystic dysplasia
- Abscess
- Tubular ectasia

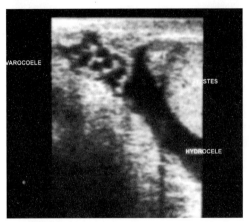

Fig. 12.4.3A: Varicocele—multiple anechoic tubular channels are seen in both the scrotal sacs

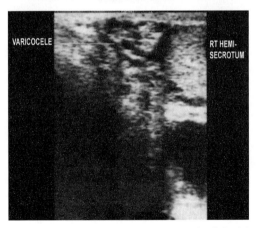

Fig. 12.4.3B: Hydrocele is seen on the left side

- Tunica albuginea cyst
- Adrenal rests
- Sarcoidosis
- Infarcts
- Calcification.

Extratesticular

- Varicocele
- Hernia
- Hemato-/Pyo-/hydrocele
- Epididymal lesions
- Tumors: Benign—adenomatoid and cystadenoma, cholesterol granuloma, soft tissue tumors.

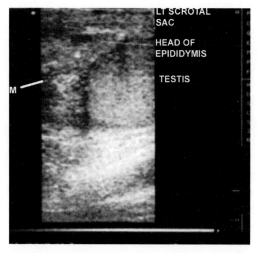

Fig. 12.4.4: A heterogeneous predominantly echogenic SOL is seen in the left scrotal sac superior to testis in a case of left inguinal hernia

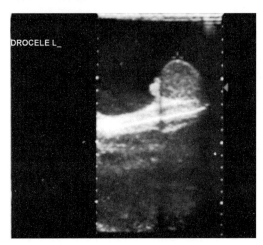

Fig. 12.4.5: Gross hydrocele

Malignant—soft tissue tumors, lymphoma, metastasis.

General Points

- Most extratesticular masses are benign while intratesticular masses should be considered malignant unless proved otherwise
- Most benign lesions are uniformly echogenic while all echogenic lesions should not be considered benign blindly
- Most malignancies are hypoechoic to normal testes unless complicated by calcification, necrosis, hemorrhage and fatty change.

Testis and Epididymis

13.1 DIFFERENTIAL DIAGNOSIS OF CYSTIC TESTICULAR LESIONS

Benign Cysts

a. Simple cyst.
b. Tubular ectasia.
c. Cystic dysplasia.
d. Abscess.
e. Tunica albuginea cyst.
f. Epidermoid cyst.

Malignant Cystic Lesions

a. Teratocarcinoma.
b. Yolk sac tumor.
c. Hemorrhage and necrosis in any mass.
d. Tubular obstruction because of any tumor.
e. Lymphoma.

Cysts in Testis are Discovered Incidentally in 8-10 percent of Population

Tunica Albuginea Cysts

- 2-5 mm, located on anterior/lateral aspect
- Simple cystic in nature

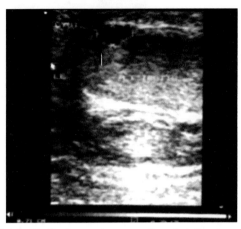

Fig. 13.1.1: Testicular cyst—a small well-defined anechoic area seen in the left testis

- 5th to 6th decades, asymptomatic
- Solitary/multiple, unilocular/multilocular.

Tubular Ectasia

- Tubular ectasia of rete testis can occur due to malignant/inflammatory traumatic obstruction of the epididymis
- Seen as multiple abnormal, tortuous channels in the region of mediastinum showing no color flow
- Usually bilateral, may be associated with ipsilateral spermatocele formation.

Cystic Dysplasia

- Congenital non-communication between tubules and rete testes/efferent ductules

- Infant and young children
- Associated with renal agenesis/dysplasia
- Multiple interconnecting simple cysts in area of rete testis extending into adjacent parenchyma, causing it atrophy.

Epidermoid Cyst

- Benign tumor of germ cell origin
- One percent of all testicular tumors
- 2nd to 4th decades of life
- Lying below tunica albuginea
- Are basically teratomas showing monomorphic, monodermal differentiation along the lines of ectodermal cell differentiation
- Present as testicular enlargement or a painless solitary nodule
- Well defined, solid, hypoechoic mass which may have internal echoes and has an echogenic capsule.

Abscess

- Looks like an abscess elsewhere and differentiation from malignancy [especially in AIDS] patients is sometimes very difficult
- May occur as a complication of epididymo-orchitis, missed testicular torsion, primary pyogenic arthritis and gangrenous/infected tumor
- Infections that may cause it are mumps, smallpox, scarlet fever, influenza, typhoid, sinusitis, osteo-myelitis, appendicitis
- May lead to pyocele formation if it rupture through tunica vaginalis or a fistula from skin.
Malignancies are considered in next topic.

13.2 PEDIATRIC TESTICULAR MASSES

- Mostly malignant
- Two peaks, i.e. 2½ yr and adolescent
- Incidence increases 30 to 50 times in a dysplastic gonad like undescended testes, male pseudohermaphroditism, true hermaphroditism, testicular feminization syndrome.
- The malignancies seen most commonly in dysplastic gonads are seminoma and gonadoblastoma due to abscence of hormonal effects
- All tumors have a non-specific USG appearance, i.e. focal/diffuse, increase/decrease echogenicity or even isoechogenicity, the size of testes may/may not increase the contour may be smooth or lobulated
- Because most lesions are isoechoic therefore altered vascularity by color Doppler is an important indicator
- Orchitis which shows similar features seldom occurs without epididymitis and is always associated with constitutional symptoms
- Simple cyst though rare may be seen
- Endodermal sinus tumor = 1-2 yr age + hernia + hydrocele + lung secondaries minus retroperitoneal lymph nodes
- Embryonal cell carcinoma = adolescent + lung metastasis + retroperitoneal lymphadenopathy.

GERM CELL TUMORS

Seminoma

Age

4th to 5th decades, rare prepuberty.

Nature

- Less aggressive than others
- Confined within tunica
- Only 25 percent metastasize at presentation
- Most favorable prognosis
- Metachronous/synchronous germ cell tumor occurs in 1-25 percent cases
- Increased incidence in a cryptorchid testes and even in a contralateral normal testes.

USG

- Well defined/ill defined
- Hypoechoic/very hypoechoic
- Homogenous
- No cyst/calcification.

Embryonal Cell Carcinoma

Age

2nd to 3rd decades, uncommon prepubertal.

Nature

- Usually in combination with others
- Aggressive, poorly radio/chemosensitive
- Visceral metastasis seen.

USG

- Inhomogenous
- Poorly marginated
- Distorts the contour, invades tunica
- Cystic area/calcification may be seen.

Endodermal Sinus/Yolk Sac Tumor

Age

- Less than two years
- Most common germ cell tumor in infants
- 60 percent of testicular tumor in infants.

Nature

- Infantile form of above.
- Increased serum AFP in 95 percent.

USG

Same as above.

Teratoma

Age

- Infancy and early childhood.

Nature

- Second peak in third decade
- Second most common testicular tumor is your
- One-third metastasize via lymphatics
- Prognosis however is fair
- In young mostly mature non-aggressive.

USG

Well defined, markedly inhomogenous with solid, cystic areas and calcification.

Choriocarcinoma

Age

Second/third decade of life.

Nature

- Rarest type, rarely occurs in pure form
- Highly malignant
- Metastasize early by hematogenous and lymphatic routes
- Symptoms referable to metastatic sites are common presenting feature like carebrovascular accident, hemoptysis
- Gynecomastia due to increased hCG.

USG

Mixed echogenicity, ill defined lesion.

Mixed Germ Cell Tumor

- Second most common testicular malignancy after seminoma
- Most common combination is one of teratoma and embryonal cell carcinoma known as terato-carcinoma.

STROMAL TUMORS

- Usually constitute of multiple cell types
- A combination with germ cell tumors also known as gonadoblastoma, occurs predominantly in males with cryptorchidism, hypospadias and female internal secondary organ

- Most common stromal tumor is Leydig cell tumor which presents at about 20 to 50 years of age as a case of painless unilateral testicular enlargement or mass
- Above is associated with impotence loss of libido or precocious virilization, gynecomastia
- Above is a small, solid, hypoechoic mass with few cystic areas.

OCCULT PRIMARY TUMORS

- Due to high metabolic rate and vascular compromise large tumors regress on their own leaving only a fibrocalcific scar, and such are known as burned out tumors.

TESTICULAR METASTASIS

- Most common testicular tumor in men over sixty years of age
- Most common bilateral testicular tumor especially malignant lymphomatous deposits
- Poor prognosis
- Homogenously hypoechoic, extending to adjacent areas and increased vascularity
- Nonlymphomatous deposits though rare come from lung, prostate, kidney, stomach, colon, pancreas, melanoma and neuroblastoma.

13.3 DIFFERENTIAL DIAGNOSIS OF EPIDYMAL LESIONS

Epididymal Cysts

- Dilated epididymal tubules

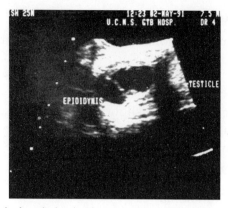

Fig. 13.3.1: Anechoic simple cyst with a thin septa seen in the region of head of the epididymis. Note the absence of internal echoes

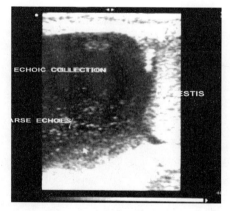

Fig. 13.3.2: A large anechoic collection with coarse internal echoes superior to left testis—spermatocele

- Result from prior epididymitis or trauma.
- Appear as simple cystic lesion.

Spermatocele

- Commoner but radiological indistinguishable from epididymal cyst
- Their location is almost always in head as against cyst that may occur in any part of epididymis
- The contents are slightly more echogenic and granular due to presence of fat, lymphocytes and spermatozoa as compared to cyst that have a simple serous content.

Sperm Granuloma

- Results after vasectomy due to extravasation of seminiferous fluid into epididymis.

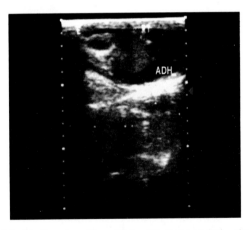

Fig. 13.3.3: Hydrocele with epididymitis (tubercular)—the epididymis is swollen and shows a hypoechoic area in it. Hydrocele shows multiple strands in it

Post-vasectomy Changes

- Enlargement of epididymis associated with heterogeneity of echotexture and formation of cysts and granuloma.

Chronic Epididymitis

- Few complex cystic lesions associated with thickened tunica and calcifications are the features.
- Associated changes in the testes may also be seen.

14

Prostate

14.1 DIFFERENTIAL DIAGNOSIS OF PROSTATIC CYST

Congenital

1. Mullerian remnant cyst.
2. Utricle cyst.

Acquired

1. Ejaculatory duct obstruction due to stone/operation.
2. Cystic change in tumors.
3. Retention cysts.
4. Benign prostatic hypertrophy.

14.2 MULLERIAN CYST

Mullerian Cyst	*Utricle Cyst*
1. Large in size.	Small in size.
2. Lateral/paramedian.	Median.
3. Has no sperms in it.	Sperms present.
4. No other associations.	Associated with renal anomalies.

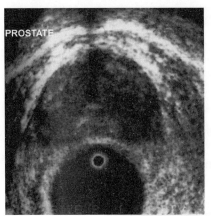

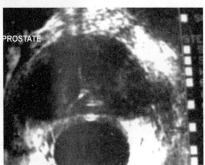

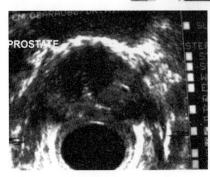

Figs 14.1.1A to C: Benign prostatic hypertrophy

14.3 EJACULATORY DUCT CYST

- Small
- Represent a diverticula or dilated obstructed duct
- Associated with infertility, perineal pain and low sperm count.

14.4 SEMINAL VESICLE CYST

- Result of wolfian duct abnormality.

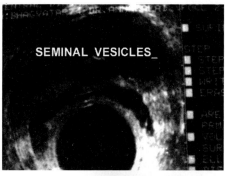

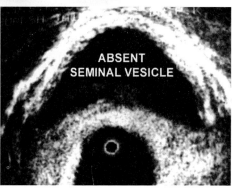

Figs 14.4.1A and B: A. Normal seminal vesicles, and B. absent seminal vesicles

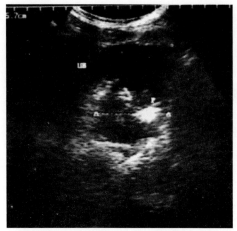

Fig. 14.4.2: Carcinoma prostate—transverse scan of prostate shows a predominantly hypoechoic enlarged prostate with a focus of calcification invading the bladder base: the interface between prostate and bladder base is lost

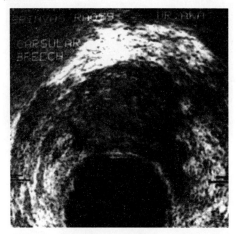

Fig. 14.4.3A: Carcinoma prostate: peripheral zone capsular invasion

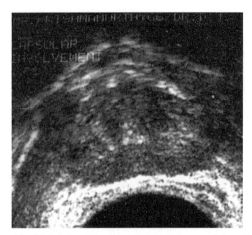

Fig. 14.4.3B: Carcinoma prostate: peripheral zone capsular invasion

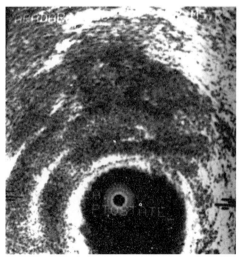

Fig. 14.4.4: Advanced carcinoma of prostate

- May be associated with ipsilateral renal agenesis, ectopic ureter and vas deferens agenesis congenital
- Usually large, unilateral, solitary
- Associated with infection, invasive bladder tumor, ejaculatory duct obstruction.

14.5 HYPOECHOIC LESIONS

- Adenocorcoma (35%)
- Benign prostatic hyperplasia (18%)—rarely may originate in peripheral zone
- Normal prostate tissue (18%)
    - i. cluster of prostate retention cysts
    - ii. prominent ejaculatory ducts
- Acute/chronic prostatitis (14%)
- Granulomatous prostatitis (10.80%)—most common due to Calmette-Guérin bacillus
- Atrophy (10%)
    - i. occurs in (70%) of young healthy men
    - ii. may be confused from carcinoma.
- Prostatic dysplasia (6%).

15

Breast

15.1 CYSTIC LESIONS

1. *Simple cysts*
   Typical appearance is—
   - Round or oval in shape

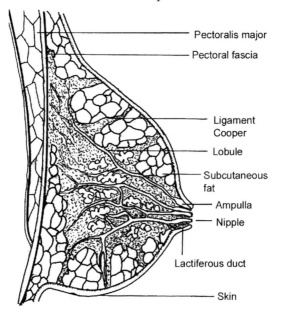

Fig. 15.1.1

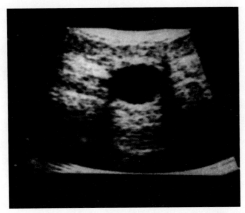

Fig. 15.1.2: A well-defined rounded systic SOL with scattered internal echoes with posterior acoustic enhancement

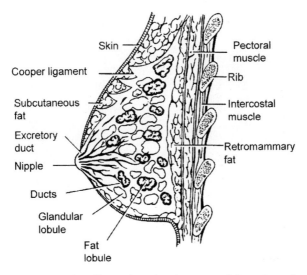

Fig. 15.1.3: Line illustration showing normal breast anatomy

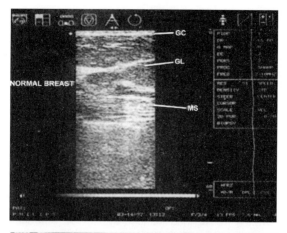

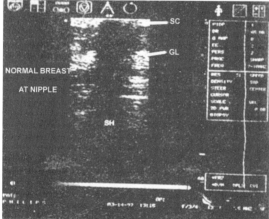

Figs 15.1.4A and B: Ultrasound of breast shows normal anatomy

- Well defined
- Smooth thin wall
- Echo free mass

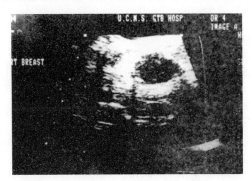

Fig. 15.1.5: Chronic abscess—right breast: US shows a well-defined hypoechoic mass with internal echoes and post-edge enhancement

- Distal enhancement
- Through transmission
- If sonographic criteria of a simple cyst are not, it is classified as a complicated cyst wherein cyst aspiration is warranted.

2. *Infected cysts*

   With fine mobile internal echoes, thick walls and surrounding edema.

   CDFI—increased low resistance vascularity surrounding the lesion

3. *Intracystic papilloma*
   - Typically, polypoidal mass is noted within the cyst with demonstrable vascularity in color doppler.

4. *Intracystic carcinomas*
   - Complicated cyst with wall irrigularity.

   Often the aspirated contents are blood stained and it reappears quickly.

5. *Oil cysts* Frequently seen in postoperative breasts.

6. *Breast abscess*
Seen as anechoic or echopoor area with diffusely increased echogenicity of the breast tissue and surrounding prominent vascularity.

7. *Subaceous cysts*
Can be echofree or contain some reflective material and even calcification.

8. *Hydatid cyst*—variable appearance on us as elsewhere in the body simple cystic appearance, rare.

9. *Filarial cyst*—a moving filarial worm (filarial dance) is a rare specific finding on realtime US.

10. *Lymphocele*—usually in post operative cases

11. *Breast prosthesis*

12. *Galactocele*—is a milk filled retention cyst during-pregnancy lactation, in newborn and infants.

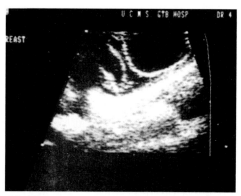

Fig. 15.1.6: Ultrasonography of left breast showing an anechoic lesion with collapsed membranes and septations—hydatid cyst

On US appears as single/multloculated cystic lesion which is easily compressible.

- Anechoic or hypoechoic (depending upon type of milk).

15.2 HYPERECHOIC LESIONS

1. *Lipomas* have echogenicity similar to the subcutaneous fat.
2. *Hemangioma*
3. *Hamartoma*—US features depend on the amount of fatty, glandular or fibrous tissue.
4. *Abscess* Typically, reveals reflective zone in the inflamed area and surrounding high vascularity.
5. Ruptured breast prosthesis with granuloma.
6. Carcinomas larger than 2 cm especially colloid carcinoma.

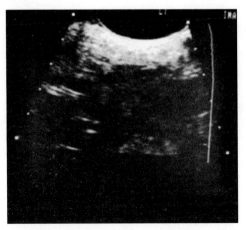

Fig. 15.2.1: Breast abscess—SOL with ill-defined margins with internal echoes in outer quadrants of left breast. Superficial fat is thickened and echogenic

7. Mastitis.
8. Hematoma—acute.
9. Angiosarcoma.

15.3 HYPOECHOIC LESIONS

Benign Lesions

1. Fibroadenoma
   • Giant fibroadenoma
   • Juvenile fibroadenoma.
2. Pseudoangiomatous stromal hyperplasia PASH
   • seen in perimenopausal women.
3. Fat necrosis.
4. Old hematoma.
5. Sclerosing adenosis.

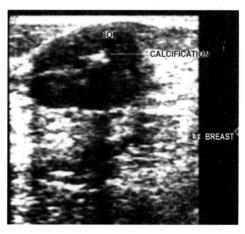

Fig. 15.3.1: Benign breast neoplasm—a well-defined homogeneously hypoechoic SOL with a dense focus of calcification

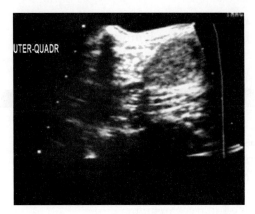

Fig. 15.3.2: Fibroadenoma—well-defined SOL of homogenous echotexture as a moblie lump in right upper outer quadrant

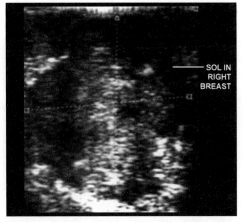

Fig. 15.3.3: Giant fibroadenoma large mass occupying most of breast with well-defined margin and slightly heterogenous echotexture

6. Radial scar.
7. Intramammary lymph node.
8. Scar granuloma.

15.4 MALIGNANT LESIONS

Principal US features are—
- Mass (nidus)
- Surrounding reflective zone (halo)
- Retrotumoral attenuation (shadow)
  1. Invassive ductal carcinoma
  2. Medullary carcinoma
  3. Sarcomas
  4. Metastasis
  5. Lymphoma
  6. Recurrent tumors.

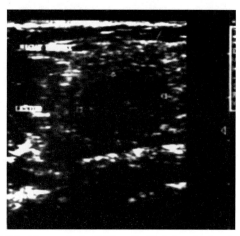

Fig. 15.4.1: Hypoechoic SOL with ill-defined lateral margins FNAC confirmed infiltrating duct carcinoma

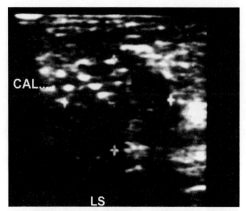

Fig. 15.4.2: Infiltrating duct carcinoma—mass calcification in breast carcinoma

15.5 DUCTAL DILATATION

1. Duct ectasia—on US, this entity is diagnosed when the duct caliber exceeds 3 mm.
2. Plasma cell mastitis.
   Minimal ductal dilatation with thick reflective walls.
3. Intraductal papilloma can occasionally be identified in the subareolar ducts smaller and peripherally located lesions are not revealed on US.
4. Ductal carcinoma *in situ* (DCIS)—sonography does not contribute to the detection of DCIS. It may reveal larger microcalcification as relatively strong echoes or dilated hypoechoic ductal structures.
5. Late pregnancy lactating breasts.

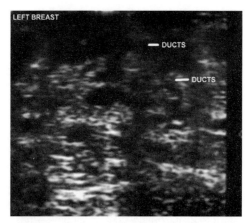

Fig. 15.5.1: Dilated ducts are seen in left breast

15.6 BENIGN VS MALIGNANT

	Beingn	*Malignant*
Shape	Oval/ellipsoid	Variable
Alignment	Wider than deep	Deeper than wide
	Aligned parallel	
	to tissue planes	
Margins	Smooth/thin echogenic	Irregular or
	pseudocapsule with	spiculated
	2-3 gentle lobulations	Echogenic 'halo'
Echotexture	Variable to intense	Markedly
	hyperechogenicity	hypoechoic
Homogeneity	Uniform	Absent
Shadowing	Present	Absent
Posterior	Minimal	Marked
enhancement		
Other signs	Coarse calcification	Fine/stippled
	macrolobulation,	calcification ,
	well defined	microlobulation,
		infiltration across
		tissue planes.

15.7 MASTITIS

Mastitis is a diffuse inflammation of the breast or a part of it. It can be infectious (usually *Staphylococcus*) and noninfections (after irridiation). On US, there is increased reflectivity of the subcutaneous fat, skin thickening which later on can progress to abscess formation. CDFI reveals increased vascularity.

Plasma cell mastitis results in focal or more generalized attenuation, with disruption of the tissue planes in the breast and thickened duct walls.

Vascular Abnormalities

Can occur in the form of solid masses as hemangiomas or cystic lesions as venous malformations.

Mondor's Disease

Mondor's disease is a thrombosed subcutaneous vein, clinically presenting as phlebitis and retraction of the skin along the track of the vein, which can be easily demonstrated on ultrasound.

Lipomas

Lipomas are common benign findings which on US appear as well delineated compressible masses with an echotexture similar to normal fat. Some lipomas have fibrous reaction due to which they are more reflective than the surrounding fat.

Sclerosing Lesions

On US, they are sharply delineated hypoechoic lesions which may show round attenuation. Examples in this category are—medial scar or sclerosing adenosis.

Hamartoma or Fibroadenolipomas

Hamartoma of breast are composed of mixture of fatty, glandular and fibrous tissue in varying amounts but fat is the permanent constituent.

Breast Prosthesis

Mammography is difficult in these cases which makes ultrasound and MRI a much popular choice for evaluating such patients. The breast tissue is located superficially to the prosthesis and therefore easily visualized.

Prosthesis is seen as an echopoor structure which is comnonly superficially with significant reverbera-tion artefacts and outer double envelope or sometimes a fibrous capsule larger fluid collections with wrin-kles of the disrupted invelope suggest ruptured prosthesis.

Gynecomastia

Refers to the condition characterized by unilateral (73%) enlargement of the glandular tissue of the breast in males which could be due to hormonal imbalance or drug induced changes. Sonographically, it can be seen as an oval shaped, well circumscribed mass or a diffuse reflective area similar to the parenchyma of an adult mature female breast.

Breast Ultrasound

15.8 BENIGN LESIONS

Cysts

• Quite common

- One quarter of the patients aged 35-50 yr
- Almost invariably, multiple and bilateral
- Calcification is infrequent, however thin peripheral eggshell may be seen
- US shows—a well defined echo-free mass with distal enhancement, round when tense and through transmission.

Variants

- Fluid level if few thickened internal contents
- Solid lesion if complete filling by thick contents in these cases, aspiration under US guidance clarifies the diagnosis
- Infectedcysts reveal fine internal echoes, thick walls and surrounding edema. On CDFI, there is increased low resistance vascularity around the infected cyst
- Intracystic papillomas—more common than the intracystic carcinomas. On US, seen as a polypoid mass within the cyst with demonstrable vascularity on color Doppler
- Intracystic carcinomas—are rare but synchronous occurrence is common. Often the aspiration contents from such a lesion is blood stained. The US sensitivity for cysts is almost 100 percent.

Fibroadenoma

It is the commonest benign tumor of breast which is thought to arise from adenosis.

- These are frequently multiple and bilateral and rarely exceed 30 mm in diameter

- They generally are seen in young females
- On US, it is demonstrated as a hypoechoic solid, well defined round or oval shaped slightly lobulated mass with uniform internal echotexture.
  Its long axis less along the tissue planes of the breast.
  Coarse calcifications in it are brightly reflective on US lesion is mobile and compressible
- Fibroadenomas classically cause displacement of the glandular tissue rather than disruption and do not have a halo around the lesion.

1. Giant fibroadenoma—is the term used for large lesion of 4 cm or more and tends to appear more in younger patients and can be more vascular.
2. Juvenile fibroadenoma—are formed in adolescents; they grow rapidly. Lesions are poorly reflective and because of the volume, may cause acoustic enhancement. These lesions are usually highly vascular, probably coresponding to then rapid growth.

Phylloides Tumor

It is uncommon, also known as 'cystosarcoma phylloides' and may appear at any age.

- On US, they are well circumscribed mass, with an oval, rounded or lobulated shape and without a halo. Slit-like fluid filled spaces when seen are diagnostic. Necrosis and hemorrhage in larger tumors may give inhomogenous echotexture.

Pseudo-angiomatous Stromal Hyperplasia (PASH)

PASH is a rare benign lesion in perimenopausal women seen as a solid, well defined poorly reflective mass similar to fibroadenoma.

Papilloma

- Usually occurs in the retro-areolar region and 35-55 year age group
- Clinically, there is serous or serosanguineous nipple discharge
- Papillomas can be intraductal, intracystic or solid like masses.

Fat Necrosis

- It is usually post-traumatic. On US, seen as markedly attenuating poorly defined echopoor masses with fluid spaces. CDFI helps in differentiating it from the carcinoma.

Oil Cysts

- These are frequently seen in postoperative breasts. US features depend on the density of the content and amount of calcification of the cyst wall.

15.9 MALIGNANT LESIONS

Invasive ductal carcinoma accounts for 80 percent of the breast carcinomas. The principal US features of a breast carcinoma are a mass, a surrounding reflective zone and retrotumoral attenuation along with often findings such as disruption of the tissue planes, skin thickening, architectural distortion and micro-calcification.

The tumor mass is poorly reflective with ill defined margins and heterogenous echotexture, if tumor is of longer size due to areas of necrosis.

Medullary carcinomas are typically well defined though not as sharply marginated as a typical fibroadenoma.

83-97 percent of carcinomas of >2 cm in diameter are attenuating which is deep to the center of the carcinoma.

Intraductal spread can sometimes be demonstrated on US.

Colloid carcinomas appear on US as a well defined lobulated mass which are highly reflective similar to the subcutaneous fat and more echogenic than other tumors.

Diffuse carcinoma—give rise to two appearances; first is in which the breast is largely replaced by poorly reflective tissue without any posterior attenuation. In these cases FNAC is required for the diagnosis. The other diffuse change occurs when there is either widespread involvement of lymphatics by cancer or following axillary dissection in which case there is breast edema. CDFI may show diffuse hyperemia.

Metastasis

Though rare but common primaries are opposite breast, lung, kidney, GIT, melanoma or hematological malignancies. The lesions are often multiple, hypoechoic, rounded and grow faster.

Lymphoma

Accounts for only 0.5 percent of all breast malignancies. Their appearances are described: first is a discrete, solitary or multiple nodular form which are hypoechoic and another is a diffuse hypoechoic enlargement of breast tissue with enlarged lymph nodes.

Local Recurrence

- Usually occurs after mastectomy or conservative surgery. Sometimes lesion occurs even after 10 yr of surgery. Lesion is often in skin or subcutaneous tissue which are seen on US as ill defined hypoechoic lesions with high vascularity.

  Fibrosis scar, which is sometimes difficult to differentiate from the recurrent tumor, is usually echogenic without a demonstrable mass or nidus and vascularity on CDFI.

  Fifty percent of all breast cancers arise in upper outer quadrant since it contains more glandular tissue than any other section of the breast. The next commonest site is retroareolar region (18%) on which ducts from the entire breast converge

1. Scar granulomas seen as hypoechoic small nodules with/without distal acoustic shadowing.
2. Silicon granulomas.
   US shows a hyperechoic masses with marked acoustic attenuation if calcified—a thin crescentic hyperechoic rim is seen to the transducer.
   - Characteristically the acoustic shadow gives a snow strom appearance (shadow if within lesion contains clearly identifiable echoes that decrease with depth.
3. Hydatid
   - Cyst with dependent echoes
   - Multiseptated, cyst within cyst
   - Complex cyst

- Calcified cyst seen as curvilinear hyperechoic scar with acoustic shadowing.
4. Harmartoma/adenofibrolipoma
   - Abnormal collection of normal parenchymal tissues found within the breast
   - Asymptomatic, detected on mammography
   - Soft palpable lesions.

US—shows however typically smooth margin, hypoechoic lesion having hyperechoic septa, pseudo-capsule best appreciated distally, lesion is compressible.

Hematoma

- H/o trauma either accidental or iatrogenic is usually present.
- US findings depend on the stage of hematoma.

Acute Hematoma

- Area of increased echogenicity with indistinct outline.
- Area of decreased echogenicity.
- Uncharacteristic architectural distortion.

With increasing age it becomes more sharply demarcated from the surrounding tissues. It appears hypoechoic, cystic with/without echogenic components.

Sarcomas

Sonographically they present as hypoechoic nodular lesion, with smooth or indistinct contour. Depending upon the tissue type tumor is soft and compressible (liposarcoma and angiosarcoma) or firm (fibrous histiocytomas and fibrosarcomas).

Central necrosis usually reveals an 'irregular hypo-echoic center. Angiosarcoma can be hyperechoic sono-graphy, hyperechogenicity representing haemorrhage.

Late Pregnancy and Lactation

Overall echogeniciy decreases, echopattern is homogeneous and the distented lectiferous ducts are seen as tubular extremely hypoechoic or anechoic structures cysts upto 7 mm in diameter.

16
Musculoskeletal System

16.1 HYPERECHOIC FOCI WITHIN THE SYNOVIUM

1. Cystal deposition (uric acid-calcium precipitates).
2. Infection (due to cellular elements and fibrin).
3. Corticosteroids (especially following recent injection).
4. Bony Fragments (in neuropathic joints).
5. Rarely in normal joint—probably related to nitrogen.

16.2 CYSTIC MASS IN POPLITEAL FOSSA

1. Popliteal cyst/Baker's cyst
   - Caused by abnormal distension of gastrocnemio-semimembranosus bursa
   - Communicates with knee joint through a slit at the posteromedial aspect of the joint capsule
   - Large cysts dissecting into the calf or ruptured cyst produce a swollen painful limb that mimics thrombophlebitis
2. Aneurysms especially popliteal artery

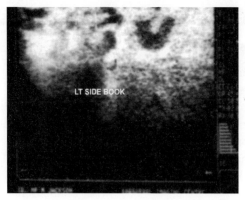

Fig. 16.2.1: US scan showing dilated vascular channels suggestive of hemangioma

- Pulsatile cystic masses with outpouching or dilatation of an artery
- CFI will settle the diagnosis
- Seen in midline or laterally.

3. Neurilemmomas
   - Seen laterally
   - Pathology establishes the diagnosis.
4. Ganglion cysts
   - (Most commonly seen at the wrist)
   - Usually midline
   - Oval fluid collection adjacent to the joint space or tender
   - Chronic cyst or cysts with viscous material may have internal echoes.
5. Adventitial cystic disease of popliteal artery.
6. Cystic appearing sarcomas, e.g. synovial sarcomas, myxoid liposarcoma.

16.3 HIP JOINT EFFUSION IN ADULTS

Causes

1. Septic arthritis.
2. Avascular necrosis.
3. Inflammatory and noninflammatory arthritis.
4. Hemorrhage, e.g. hemophilia and other bleeding disorders.
5. Tumors as pigmented villonodular synovitis and synovial osteochondromatosis.

16.4 PROLIFERATIVE SYNOVITIS

1. Rheumatoid arthritis.
2. Septic arthritis (a) acute: bacterial, (b) subacute: tumberculosis, fungal, etc.
3. Crystal induced arthropathies.
4. Amyloid arthropathy.
5. Pigmented villonodular synovitis.
6. Synovial osteochondromatosis.
7. Hemophillic arthropathy.

16.5 TENDON TEARS

Signs

Partial tear

1. Discontinuity of some fibers.
2. Acute tear appears as hypoechoic defect in tendon.

Complete tear

- Discontinuity of all fibers.
- Nonvisualisation of retracted tendon.
- Hematoma, usually

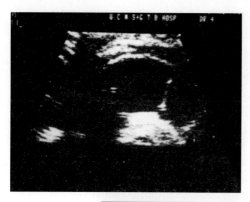

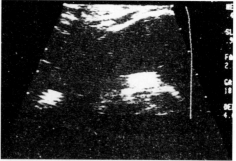

Figs 16.5.1A and B: Sagittal and transverse scans of right shoulder showing break in continuity of rotator cuff

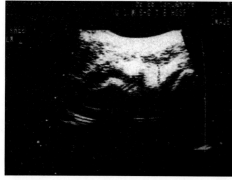

Fig. 16.5.2: US of the right knee showing linear hypoechoic area—tear (arrow) in posterior horn of lateral meniscus

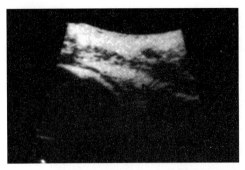

Fig. 16.5.3: US—sagittal view showing hypoechoic area (arrow) within homogenicity of echotexture of posterior horn of medial meniscus suggestive of mensical tear

3. Hematoma, usually very small.

small.
- Bone fragment in case of bone avulsion.

Partial tear needs to be differentiated from focal tendinitis.

Signs of Tendinitis

1. Thickening of the tendon.
2. Decreased echogenicity.
3. Blurred margins.
4. Increased vascularity on CFI.
5. Calcification in chronic cases.

USG—Findings in Proliferative Synovitis

1. Hypoechogenicity and thickening of synovial membrane often with irregularity and nodularity.
2. Hyperechogenicity of fat adjacent to inflamed synovium.
3. Effusion in joint cavity.

16.6 PEDIATRIC HIP JOINT—AN OVERVIEW

The most important determinant of the outcome of an infected hip is the delay between the onset and treatment. Conventional radiographic examinations are of little help in early diagnosis. Computed tomography and MRI though informative are very expensive and not universally available. With ultrasound (US) scanning even small fluids/pus collections of 1-2 ml can be accurately detected. The use of other (invasive) imaging modalities can be minimised as US can be used to demonstrate effusions early in the disease along with the status of the intra-articular compartment, joint capsule, bony surface and adjacent soft tissues. US scanning should be used more commonly to diagnose infective arthritis and no patient should be subjected to arthrotomy or drainage, if US scan has ruled out the presence of a fluid collection. Over last one decade sonography of hip has been used in the diagnosis of congenital dislocation, or dysplasia and Perthes' disease. US scan well demonstrates the soft tissue structures around hip and unossified cartilage without any radiation and pain. Arthrography though useful, is painful, requires anesthesia and injection of contrast. The sonography can suggest dysplasia/dislocation by presence of rounded deformed head, loss of concavity, inclination of acetabular roof, lateralization, delayed ossification center and percentage of coverage. The sonography in Perthes' disease can define the irregu-larity of femoral head and rate of deformity of the same. The purpose of writing this overview is to highlight the usefulness of US scanning to diagnose various hip disorders in children accurately and quickly.

With development of high-resolution realtime transducers, ultrasound (US) scanning has become the investigation of choice in the initial evaluation of hip joint in children. With US scanning, direct imaging of even the unossified parts is also possible. Presence of synovitis and effusion, development of head of femur, acetabulum and their anatomical interrelationship can be sonographically assessed without any risk of radiation and contrast.

Joint Effusion and Infective Arthritis

Pain, refusal to bear weight and limping can be due to a wide variety of conditions affecting the hip joint. Clinically, it is difficult many times to differentiate between the intrinsic abnormality and the pseudo

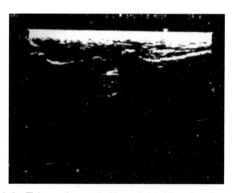

Fig. 16.6.1: Tubercular arthritis—right hip showing increased anterior synovial recess with convex and anechoic collection. Left hip is normal

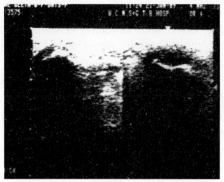

Fig. 16.6.2: Pyogenic arthritis—left hip showing destruction of femoral head. The anterior synovial recess is widened with echogenic collection. Right hip is normal

flexion deformity of the joint. The plain films are both insensitive and unreliable in their diagnosis. Though computed tomography (CT) may be more informative, US provides an easily available, quick and accurate noninvasive technique to detect intra-articular abnormalities. Extra-articular pathologies like pelvic abscess, appendicitis, iliac lymphadenitis and osteomyelitis can also be diagnosed and differentiated from intra-articular pathology although clinical presentation may be similar.

Technique

The patient is examined in the supine position using 4-7.5 MHz linear/sector realtime transducer. Anterior longitudinal approach along the neck femur is the simple, most useful imaging plane. Both hips are examined in every case.

Normal sonographic anatomy reveals the following:

1. Joint capsule is seen as a liner echnogenic band like structure (2 mm thick) anteriorly, along the contour of head and neck. The band extends from acetabular rim to its insertion at intertrochanteric line.
2. Anterior synovial recess is seen as a 3 mm wide clear space between capsule and bony surface.
3. Growth plate.
4. Surrounding soft tissue, ileopsoas muscle and pelvis.

Abnormal Hip

The affected hip may show collection in anterior synovial recess more than 3 mm width and with an asymmetry of at least 2 mm on both sides. Echo pattern of synovial fluid in septic hip may show hyper-echoic character due to high cellular content or bleeding. Tubercular arthritis, transient synovitis and treated septic arthritis may show hypoechoic synovial collection but varied picture is present as hyperechoic character though less common has been observed in transient synovitis and tubercular arthritis. The positive predictivity of US for diagnosing effusion in our experience is over 95%. The capsule may show thickening and anterior bulge. The convex contour suggests raised intra-articular pressure which can interfere with blood supply to head and any delay in institution of therapy can result in irreversible changes. Surgical arthrotomy/ US guided aspiration can now be easily done to relieve the pressure and establish the etiological diagnosis. There has been a marked drop in negative arthrotomy at our institution since the use of sonography in evaluation of hip joint. Minimal collections under conservative management and postoperative cases can be monitored sonographically to follow the course of the disease process.

Perthes' Disease

Frequent measurements of growth and development of femur head are essential in these patients to monitor the course of disease. The head should retain its sphericity along with its growth for best functional utility. Many radiographic methods have been developed for this assessment. Precise assessment is not possible with these methods if the child is young and cartilaginous parts are not visible or arthrography is required, which is a painful procedure needing general anesthesia, radiation and injection of contrast.

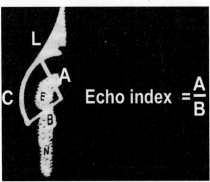

Fig. 16.6.3: Sketch diagram seen in lateral coronal plane with adduction at hip: A—acetabulum, L—labrum, C—capsule, E—epiphysis, and N—neck femur

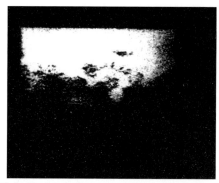

Fig. 16.6.4: Perthes' disease—lateral sonogram demonstrating the flattening head with good cartilaginous covering

US has been used to replace earlier radiographic methods, including arthrography to measure the sphericity of femur head and to determine the rate of deformity due to LCP. US can directly, noninvasively, visualize the bony and cartilaginous parts of the head.

Technique

The patient is examined in supine position with leg abducted at hip by about 35°. This maneuver allows almost lateral 2/3rd of head to be visualized. A 4-7.5 MHz transducer is placed laterally in transverse (axial) and longitudinal (coronal) planes. In the axial plane the maximum transverse diameter of head is measured. The longitudinal projections show the acetabulum, labrum, capsule, head of femur, epiphysis and growth plate. The maximum height of head from growth plate (A) and maximum width of head (B) at level of growth plate are measured. The ratio of A to B is the Echo

Index (EI). The ratio of EI of affected side to normal is defined as Echo Quotient (EQ). The EQ represents the grade of the cartilaginous femur head deformity and this facilitates follow up correlation in LCP with objective measurements over a prolonged time period. Apart from this, flattening and fragmentation of cartilaginous parts scan also be diagnosed with US scanning. To conclude, US scanning can be used in place of arthrography and radiography to determine the sphericity of femur head in LCP disease.

Congenital Dislocation and Dysplasia of LCP

In congenital dislocation of hip an early diagnosis and treatment are essential for proper development. In newborn and infant the entire proximal femur head and greater trochanter are cartilaginous. Only portions of acetabulum may be ossified. The development of these important unossified structures in hip joint can, therefore, only be assessed indirectly with X-ray

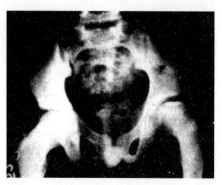

Fig. 16.6.5: AP radiograph of the same patient

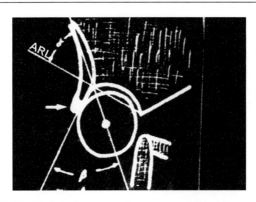

Fig. 16.6.6: Sketch diagrammatic representation of coronal sonography in infant hip—showing base line (BL), acetabular roof line (ARL) and inclination line (IL), a and b-angles

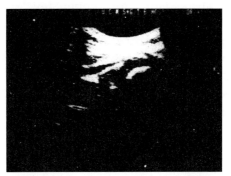

Fig. 16.6.7: Tangential lines along the femur head to measure percentage of coverage

radiographs and CT scanning or directly by invasive arthrography.

With improvement in technology of high resolution small parts transducer, sonography can directly visualize both the cartilaginous and bony parts of hip

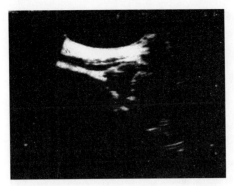

Fig. 16.6.8: Lateral sonogram of left hip showing concentric relationship of head to acetabulum and triradiate cartilage

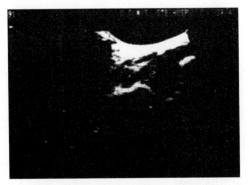

Fig. 16.6.9: Same patient's right hip showing displaced head

for accurate assessment of its size, shape and symmetry. The radiation free (US) technique is more reliable than radiography or CT scanning. The US scanning is preferred over arthrography for evaluation of infant hip due to its noninvasive nature.

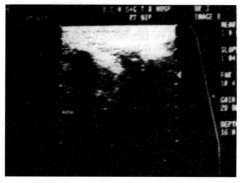

Fig. 16.6.10: Lateral sonogram of right hip showing empty acetabulum suggestive of complete dislocation of head

With realtime US scanning, dynamic studies are also possible to detect laxity of the ligamentous structures in potentially dislocated hips. Apart from establishing the diagnosis, this technique can be used to monitor the effect of treatment by repetitive studies even when the patient is in spica cast.

The main indications for performing sonography is an abnormal hip are:

i. To determine the position and development of femur head.

ii. To diagnose instability during dynamic studies with lap movements in various positions.

iii. To assess the development of acetabulum, especially the cartilaginous component.

Technique and Normal Anatomy

Both linear and sector transducer from 3-7.5 MHz frequency may be used. Higher frequency is required for neonates and lower frequency for the older patients. The patient is examined in supine position in lateral coronal and transverse planes with the transducer at greater trochanter. The plane of interest should out line the head, neck of femur, iliac bone, acetabulum, greater trochanter and joint capsule.

In lateral coronal approach the head can be seen within the acetabulum with echogenic bony ileum superiorly. The joint capsule is identified as an echogenic band surrounding the head. The acetabulum labrum is seen as a triangular structure at the edge of bony acetabulum as a hypoechoic structure. Rest of acetabular echoes are seen superiorly and medially with a gap in bony echoes due to posterior limb of triradiate cartilage.

Table 16.6.1: Classification of hip dysplasia on the basis of ultrasonographic measurements

Character	Type I (Normal)	Type II (Dysplasia)	Type III (Subluxation)
a-Angle	>60°	44 –60°	<43°
b-Angle	<55°	55 –77°	>77°
Percentage coverage	>58°	58 –33°	<33°

In transverse neutral plane the cartilaginous head is seen within the acetabulum over the central triadiate cartilage. The triadiate cartilage allows the onward transmission of sound, producing a zone of acoustic shadowing. In transverse flexion projection, the echogenic structures combine to produce a 'U' configuration with vertical limb of triradiate cartilage at its base. Anterior limb of 'U' is due to junction of metaphysis and epiphysis while posterior limb is due to echoes from acetabulum.

The objective assessment of acetabular development can be done by two methods. The first described by Graf (1984) is based on various angles formed by 3 lines:

1. Baseline (A) which connects the osseous acetabulum convexity to the point where joint capsule and perichondrium unite with iliac bone.
2. The inclination line (a) which connects the osseous convexity to labrum acetabulare.
3. The acetabular roof line (b) connecting the lower edge of ileum to osseous convexity.

Alpha Angle

This is the most important measurement and lies between base line and acetabular roof line. This angle indicates the formation of acetabular convexity.

Beta Angle

It measures the formation and development of cartilage convexity and lies between inclination line. And base line.

On the basis of these lines and angles, the hip can be classified as follows:

Type I (Normal) a angle more than 60° and b less than 55°.

Type II (Dysplasia) Includes cases of subluxation which sometimes get corrected without treatment (Delayed ossification). A angle less than 43°–60° and b between 50°–77°.

Type III The cartilaginous edges pushed outwards and upwards by the laxating femur head. a angle less than 43° and b angle more than 77°. The echo free cartilaginous head becomes echodense.

Type IV The femur head is completely dislocated into an empty acetabulum. The deformed cartilaginous edge with flat osseous edge is seen.

A relatively simple method for acetabular assessment by measuring the relative percentage of coverage of the femur head by bony acetabulum has been described. US scanning of the hip joint by lateral approach in coronal view is similar to AP radiograph and has been correlated with radiograph and has been correlated with radiographic acetabular index. The linear echogenic straight ileum echo is called iliac line, which when extended through the head, normally divides it into two parts. Two lines tangential to femur head at its medial and lateral border and parallel to iliac line are also drawn. The distance between two tangent line is 'D' and distance between iliac line and medial line is referred to as 'd'. The ratio of D: d × 100 indicates the percentage of femur head coverage by bony acetabulum. When this is correlated with acetabular index measurements made on radiography, a coverage of less than 33% is definitely abnormal and indicates dysplasia, a coverage between 33-58% is the transition zone and coverage of femoral head above 58% is normal. Follow up of patients on treatment can be made by objective serial measurements of coverage percentage.

Abnormal Hip

A small ossific nucleus may be seen as an echogenic focus with the cartilaginous head between 1-6 months of age. The ossification centre is sonographically detected earlier compared to X-ray radiography. It is often delayed in congenital dislocation of hip on the affected side.

Apart from angle measurements mentioned earlier, in dislocation the concentric relationship of the femur head to triradiate cartilage will also be seen. Lateral displacement is seen as a gap between the head and acetabular roof. In posterior and superior dislocation, head is often seen against bony ileum, without any gap. In transverse flexion the 'U' configuration of the head may be laterally positioned limb of 'U'. When there is subluxation, the femur head is often covered by the thickened stretched joint capsule and the posterior part of bony acetabulum is flatter than normal. Children with frank dislocation of hip have a very thick capsule and an abnormally small acetabulum. The head will not be seated within the acetabulum but displaced in surrounding soft tissues. With movement of limb from adduction to extreme abduction, reduction can be seen to occur in an unstable hip.

With advancement of age, US scanning becomes more difficult but is still practical till 2 years of age.

The ossification centre of more than 10 mm can also interfere with proper evaluation. Caution must be observed in very young infants with dysplasia as many unstable hips may recover spontaneously in Ist week of life.

Finally, with experience sonographic anatomy and various abnormalities of hip joints can be diagnosed with US scanning. This technique should be extensively used for assessment of the paediatric hip joint.

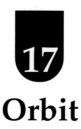

Orbit

Sonographic Classification of Orbital Lesions

- Except muscles, nerves and vitreous all normal orbital structures are hyperechoic
- Pathologies are usually hypoechoic apart few which are hyperechoic but not as much as the normal

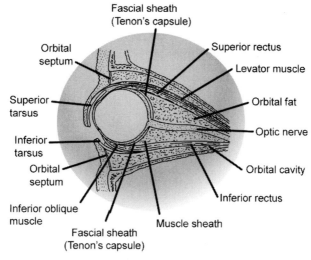

Fig. 17.1.1: Vertical section of the eye and orbit

orbital structures. Also the pathologies are heterogenous.

Extremely Low Reflectivity Lesions

1. Cysts.
2. Mucocele (Non-compressible).
3. Hematoma.
4. Varix (alters shape with Valsalva).
5. Paranasal sinus malignancy (has bony chips in it).

17.2 LOW REFLECTIVITY LESIONS

1. Cellulitis, abscess, pseudotumor.
2. Lymphoma.
3. Glioma.
4. Capillary hemangioma.
5. Caroticocavernous fistula.

17.3 MEDIUM REFLECTIVITY LESIONS

1. Dermoid.
2. Meningioma.

17.4 HIGH REFLECTIVITY LESIONS

1. Metastases.
2. Foreign Body.
3. Cavernous hemangioma.
4. Lymphangioma.
5. Pleomorphic adenoma.
   - *Pathologies may also be classified according to their edge definition.*

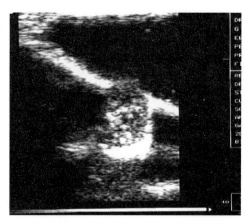

Fig.17.5.1: Epidermoid cyst—a large SOL with predominant cystic areas with internal debris is seen anterosuperiorly to the eyeball. The lesion is seen to extend intracranially and causing bone destruction. The intracranial part is predominantly solid with foci of calcification in it. The eyeball is not involved. FNAC confirmed the case

17.5 WELL CIRCUMSCRIBED MASSES/LESIONS

1. Cavernous hemangiomas.
2. Hemangiopericytomas.
3. Dermoids.
4. Meningioma.
5. Foreign body.
6. Nerve sheath tumors.

17.6 INFILTRATIVE LESIONS

1. Pseudotumor.
2. Lymphoma.
3. Metastases.

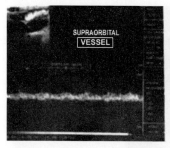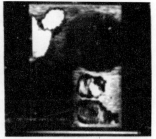

Fig.17.7.1: There is evidence of dilatation of superior ophthalmic vein and dilated vessels in the superorbital region and within extraconal compartment. The dilated vessels on duplex showed a mixed arteriovenous turbulent signal

4. Capillary hemangioma.
5. Lymphangioma.
6. Wegener's granulomatosis.

17.7 SERPINGENOUS LESIONS

1. Arterio-venous malformation.
2. Varix.
3. Plexiform neurofibroma.

17.8 DIFFERENTIAL DIAGNOSIS OF ORBITAL MUSCLE ENLARGEMENT

1. Graves' disease
   - Look for thyroid
   - Look for thyroid function tests.
2. Myositis/pseudotumor
   - Look for signs of inflammation.
3. Lymphoma.
4. Leukemia.

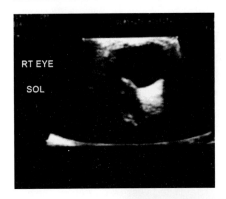

Figs17.8.1A and B: Pseudotumor—(A) longitudinal, (B) transverse scan shows well-defined, spindle shaped hypoechoic solid mass with foci of calcification in the lateral rectus muscle

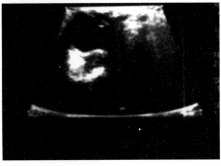

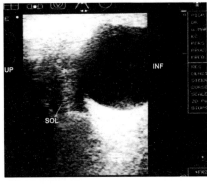

Fig.17.8.2: Follow-up case of Hodgkin's lymphoma showing a well-defined round hypoechoic SOL adjacent to the eyeball FNAC—confirmed lymphomatous origin

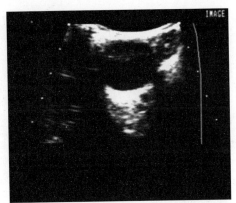

Fig.17.8.3: Orbital cysticercosis—a well-defined round cystic SOL with focus of calcification seen in muscle adjacent to eyeball

5. Metastasis.
6. Rhabdomyosarcoma/myoma.
7. Hemangioma.
8. Lymphangioma.
9. Caroticocavernous fistula.
10. Dural AVM.
11. Injury/hematoma.
12. Acromegaly.
13. Infective cysticercosis.

17.9 DIFFERENTIAL DIAGNOSIS OF U/L PROPTOSIS

Lesions of Eyeball

- Retinoblastoma:
  - Echogenic
  - Calcification present, coarse
  - Associated with retinal detachment

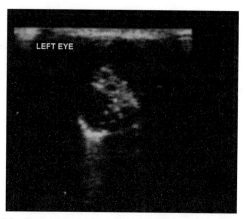

Fig.17.9.1A: Retinoblastoma—6-month-old male child showing a heterogenous echotexture mass in the left eye with multiple dense echogenic and anechoic areas

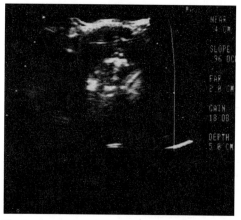

Fig.17.9.1B: Retinoblastoma—transverse scan of left eye in a 3-year-old female child showing a solid intraocular mass attached posteriorly with areas of calcification in it

- Melanoma:
  - Iso to hypoechoic
  - Adults
  - May breech the Tenon's capsule.
- Metastasis
- Hematoma
- Episcleritis
- Scleritis
- Uveitis.

Lesions of Optic Nerve

- Glioma:
  - Thickened optic nerve, focally.
  - Protruding optic disc.
- Meningioma:
  - Thickened nerve shadow but smoothly.

Lesions of Extraocular Muscles

- Myositis
- Graves' disease:
  - Increased intraorbital echogenic fat.
  - May be associated with muscle thickening.
  - No fat stranding.
- Rhadomyoma/sarcoma
- Hemangioma
- Trauma
- Lymphoma
- Leukemia.

Lesions of Lacrimal Glands

- Dacryoadenitis:
  - Bulky lacrimal glands
  - Edema in surrounding tissues.

- Lymphoma
- Mucoepidermoid tumor
- Adenoid cystic tumor
- Pleomorphic adenoma
- Sarcoidosis
- Benign cysts.

Other Intrachoanal Space Occupying Lesions

- Fibroma
- Hemangioma
- Lymphangioma
- Lipoma/sarcoma
- Lymphoma
- Varix
- Neurofibroma
- Abscess
- Hydatid
- Granuloma.

Extrachoanal Lesions

- Fibrous dysplasia
- Non-ossifying fibroma
- Subperiosteal abscess:
  - Extracoanal fluid
          (heterogenous collection)
  - Broad based towards bone.
- Mucocele.
- Carcinoma maxilla/sino-nasal malignancies
- Hematoma
- Orbital cellulitis
- Aneurysmal bone cysts.
- Epidermoid/dermoid
- Osteomyelitis.

17.10 DIFFERENTIAL DIAGNOSIS OF B/L PROPTOSIS

1. Graves' disease:
   - Intraorbital fat.
   - Abnormal thyroid function tests.
2. Metastasis
3. Lymphoma/Sarcoma:
   - Diffuse infiltrative hypoechoic lesion involving both intra and extracoanal structures.
4. Leukemia.
5. Histiocytosis.
6. Late phase of cavernous sinus thrombosis.
7. Developmental lesions of skul:
   a. Oxycephaly.
   b. Apert's syndrome.
   c. Cruzon's syndrome.

17.11 DIFFERENTIAL DIAGNOSIS OF PULSATILE PROPTOSIS

1. Caroticocavernous fistula:
   - Serpigenous tortuous hypoechoic vascular structures showing flow towards orbit are seen
   - Wave forms are one of arterialized veins.
2. Arteriovascular malformations
3. Aneurysms
4. Varix: Avascular channel that inflates on Valsalva is seen.
5. Cephalocele.
6. Neurofibromatosis with sphenoid wing dysplasia.
7. Base of skull fracture.

18

Neonatal and Infant Brain

18.1 CYSTIC LESIONS

1. Porencephalic cyst.
2. Hydranencephaly.
3. Cystic encephalomalacia.

Ventriculomegaly

1. Hydrocephalus.
2. Atrophy.
3. Colpocephaly.

Congenital/Developmental Malformations

1. Holoprosencephaly.
2. Schizencephaly.
3. Dandy-Walker malformation.
4. Arachnoid cyst.
5. Midline interhemispheric cyst.
6. Meg a cisterna magna.
7. Choroid plexus cyst.
8. Subependymal cyst.

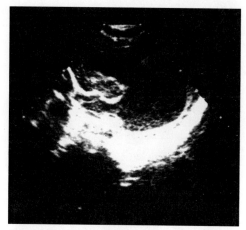

Fig. 18.1.1: Semilobar holoprosencephaly

Infections

1. Abscess.
2. Subdural effusion.
3. Empyema.

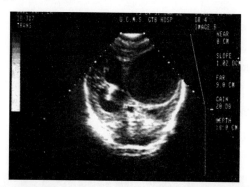

Fig. 18.1.2: Anechoic lesion in left parietal region
compressing lateral and third ventricles—brain abscess

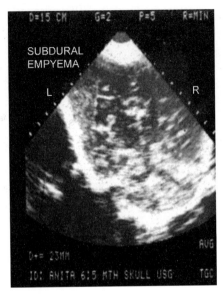

Fig. 18.1.3: Brightly echogenic meninges seen overlying the left frontal lobe with extraaxial collection containing echoes overlying it—subdural empyema

Vascular

1. Vein of Galen malformation.
2. Varix of vein of Galen.
3. AV malformation.

Trauma

1. Leptomeningeal cyst.
2. Chronic hematoma.

18.2 SOLID LESIONS

1. Intracranial hemorrhage.

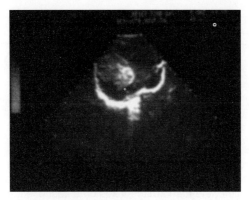

Fig. 18.2.1A: Intracranial hemorrhage in right parietal area—longitudinal and sagittal scan

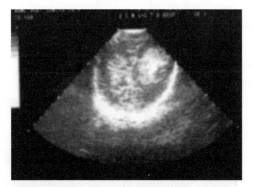

Fig. 18.2.1B: Intracranial hemorrhage in left cerebral hemisphere parietal area

2. Asphyxia.
3. Infection (cerebritis and edema).
4. Tumors.

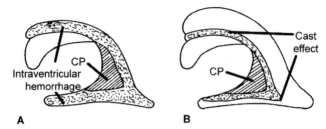

Fig. 18.3.1: Intraventricular hemorrhage. A. Lateral sagittal view. An intraventricular hemorrhage fills the entire lateral ventricle. the choroid plexus is difficult to distinguish from the hemorrhage B. With time, the hemorrhage takes on a cast effect and adopts the shape of the ventricle as the blood resolves. The choroid plexus is still difficult to distinguish from the clot

18.3 PROMINENT CHOROID PLEXUS

1. Intraventricular hemorrhage.
2. Infection.
3. Choroid plexus papilloma.

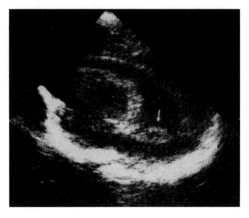

Fig. 18.3.2: Intraventricular hemorrhage (IVH)

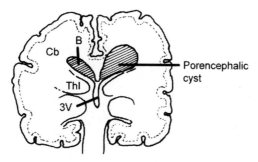

Fig. 18.4.1: The clot resolves completely, leaving a porencephalic cyst with lateral ventricular dilatation

18.4 DESTRUCTIVE LESIONS OF BRAIN

Porencephalic Cyst

- It is an area of normally developed brain that has been damaged and heals with a lining of gliotic white matter
- It is seen as a cystic area which connects to ventricular system but does not extend to surface cortex
- Typically occurs after birth as a sequelae to hemorrhage, infection and trauma.

Hydranencephaly

- Result of occlusion of bilateral internal carotid arteries in fetal life
- Regarded as severest form of porencephaly
- USG shows calvarium filled with CSF with total destruction of cerebral cortex and falx cerebri is preserved

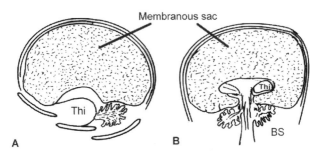

Fig. 18.4.2: A. Hydranencephaly. Lateral sagittal (A) and midcoronal (B) views. There is no evidence of cortical tissue. A membranous fluid-filled sac replaces the brain. Only the brainstem and midbrain are present

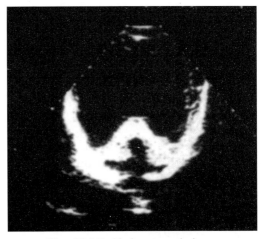

Fig. 18.4.3: Hydranencephaly

- Structures supplied by posterior circulation are spared, e.g. thalamus, cerebellum, brainstem and posterior choroid plexus.

- Doppler USG shows absence of blood flow in carotid arteries
- D/D—alobar holoprosencephaly and hydrocephalus

Differentiating Features

- Alobar holoprosencephaly
- Falx cerebri is absent in this but present in hydrancephaly
- Hydrocephalus: A thin rim of cortex is usually seen by sonography which is absent in Hydranencephaly.

Cystic Encephalomalacia

- Is an area of focal or widespread brain damage with astrocytic proliferation and glial septations
- May result from infection, anoxia and thrombus in neonatal brain

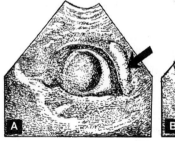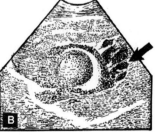

Fig. 18.4.4: Periventricular leukomalacia. A. An echogenic area surrounds the trigone of the lateral ventricle in its early stages (arrow). B. Tiny cysts develop soon afterward to replace this echogenic area (arrow)

- D/D—Porencephalic cyst.

Porencephalic cyst	Cystic encephalomalacia
Always connect with the system	Typically do not ventricular connect to ventricular system
Do not extend to surface cortex	May extend to surface cortex

18.5 VENTRICULOMEGALY

Hydrocephalus

- Enlargement of ventricles with decreased sulcal and cisternal space is identified as hydrocephalus. Imaging findings are:
  a. Enlargement of 3rd ventricle especially anterior and posterior recesses.
  b. Proportionate dilatation of the temporal horns with the lateral ventricle.
  c. Narrowing of mammilopontine distance.
  d. Narrowing of ventricular angle.
  e. Widening of frontal horn radius.
  f. Periventricular interstitial edema.
  g. Effacement of cortical sulci.

Causes of Hydrocephalus

Intraventricular obstruction	Extraventricular obstruction	Over production
Posthemorrhagic Post fossa subdural hematoma	Post hemorrhagic Post infectious	Choroid plexus papilloma

Contd...

Table contd...

Chiari II malformation	Achondroplasia
Aqueductal stenosis	— Absence or
Post infectious	hypoplasia of
Vein of Galen	arachnoid
malformation	granulation
Tumor or cyst	Venous obstruction

Sonography is Useful for

1. Diagnosis of hydrocephalus
   - Can be diagnosed *in utero* by 15 weeks of gestation
   - *In utero*, size of atrium >10 mm indicates ventriculomegaly
   - Progressive roundening and bulging of superolateral angles of frontal horns.
   - Dilatation of occipital horns.
2. Level of obstruction
   - Site of obstruction in hydrocephalus is the point of transition from dilated to nondilated CSF containing spaces, e.g.

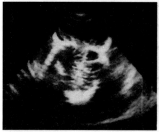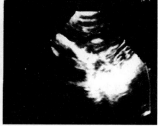

Figs 18.5.1A and B: Arnold-Chiari malformation II is showing tonsillar herniation with downward shift of fourth ventricle

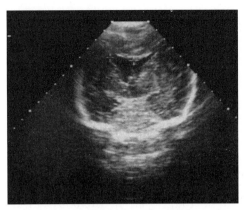

Fig. 18.5.2: Frontal horn of right lateral ventricles appears dilated. Left is normal suggestive of asymmetrical hydrocephalus due to obstruction at foramen of Monro

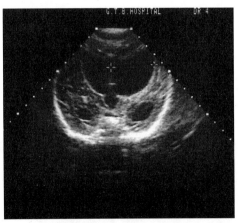

Fig. 18.5.3: Congenital aqueductal stenosis—bilateral lateral ventricles appear dilated with funnel shaped third ventricle

— Dilatation of lateral and IIIrd ventricles indicates aqueductal obstruction.

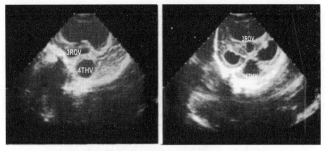

Fig. 18.5.4: Communicating hydrocephalus

— Dilatation of all ventricles indicats an extra-ventricular cause.
3. Cause of hydrocephalus
   • Presence of hemorrhage, ventriculitis is evident by intraparenchymal changes and intraventricular echoes and septations with irregular ependymal outline
   • Other well defined conditions associated with obstructive hydrocephalus, e.g. Dandy-Walker syndrome and Chiari II malformation are apparent on US.

Ventriculomegaly Secondary to Atrophy

1. There is prominence of ventricles as well as CSF spaces.
2. Small or diminishing head circumference favors atrophy.
3. Anterior and posterior recesses of 3rd ventricle are not enlarged in atrophy whereas they are enlarged in case of hydrocephalus.

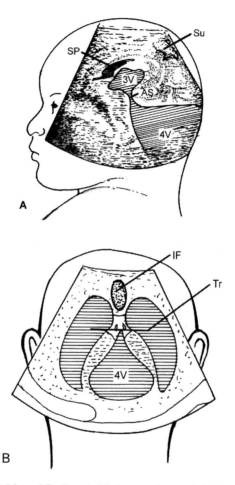

Figs 18.5.5A and B: Dandy-Walker syndrome. A. Midline sagittal view. There is cystic dilatation of the fourth ventricle; the third ventricle and aqueduct of Sylvius are dilated to some degree. Note the abnormal cerebellar shape. B. Posterior coronal view: Massive IVth ventricular and lateral ventricular enlargement

4. Temporal horns dilate less than the bodies of lateral ventricles in case of atrophy due to relatively small size of temporal lobes.

Colpocephaly

- Atria and occipital horns of lateral ventricles are disproportionately enlarged
- It is associated with Chiari II malformation and corpus callosum agenesis.

18.6 CONGENITAL AND DEVELOPMENTAL MALFORMATIONS

Holoprosencephaly

Can be alobar, semilobar or lobar types.

Sonographic Findings in Alobar Holoprosencephaly

1. Single midline crescent shaped ventricle.
2. Thin layer of cerebral cortex.

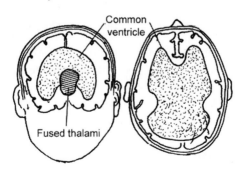

Fig. 18.6.1: Holoprosencephaly. Anterior coronal and axial views. A single misshaped ventricle is present

3. No falx.
4. No interhemispheric fissure.
5. No corpus callosum.
6. Fused thalami and basal ganglia.
7. Fused echogenic choroid plexus.
8. Absent third ventricle.
9. Large dorsal cyst.
10. Severe facial anomalies-colpocephaly, cyclopia, ethmocephaly.

Sonographic Findings in Semilobar Holoprosencephaly

1. Single ventricle but separate occipital and temporal horns.
2. Partially developed falx and interhemispheric fissure in the occipital cortex posteriorly.
3. Partially separated thalami.
4. Rudimentary 3rd ventricle.
5. Facial anomalies are less severe—hypotelorism, cleft lip.

Sonographic Findings in Lobar Holoprosencephaly

1. Nearly complete separation of hemispheres with development of falx and interhemispheric fissure but part of frontal lobes may be fused anteriorly.
2. Genu and rostrum of corpus callosum is absent.
3. Mild or absent facial anomalies.

Schizencephaly

1. Caused by a destructive process *in utero* leading to gray matter lined clefts that extend through the

entire hemisphere from ependymal lining of lateral ventricles to cortical surface.

2. B/L or U/L clefts.
3. It can be open lip type or closed lip type. Closed lip type is identified by a nipple like protrusion on the ventricular surface.

Arachnoid Cyst

1. It is seen as an cystic extraxial lesion producing mass effect with displacement of underlying brain parenchyma.
2. Does not communicate with ventricular system.

Mega Cisterna Magna

1. *In utero* mega cisterna magna is diagnosed when its AP dimension measures 5 ± 3 mm.
2. It arches around cerebellum posteriorly and is usually widest in the midline where invagination of space occurs between the two cerebellar hemispheres.
3. Not associated with hydrocephalus or abnormal brain parenchyma.

Choroid Plexus Cyst

1. Cystic well defined mass within the choroid plexus measuring 4-7 mm in diameter.
2. Usually U/L, occurring more frequently on the left and situated in the dorsal aspect of choroid plexus.
3. Rarely can cause obstructive hydrocephalus.

Subependymal Cyst

1. Discrete cysts in the lining of ventricles.
2. Commonly result from germinal matrix hemorrhage in premature infants, also due to infection with rubella, CMV and Zellweger's syndrome.

Dorsal Interhemispheric Cyst

1. Well defined anechoic cystic structure in dorsal interhemispheric fissure.
2. Associated with corpus callosum agenesis, Dandy-Walker malformation and holoprosencephaly.

Cavum Septum Pellucidum and Cavum Vergae

1. Anterior to the foramen of Monro is the cavum septum pellucidum and posterior is the cavum vergae.

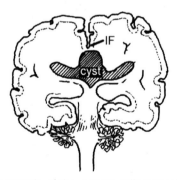

Fig. 18.6.2: Agenesis of the corpus callosum with cyst. In this variant, the lateral and third ventricles are joined by a cyst that extends superiorly from the third ventricle

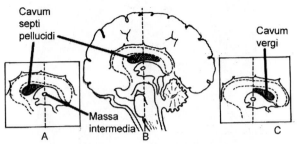

Fig. 18.6.3: Cavum septi pellucidi. If the scanning angle is incorrect, this normal variant may be mistaken for a dilated ventricle. It may appear in one of three different patterns: A. Cavum septi pellucidi. B. Cavum septi pellucidi and cavum vergae. C. Cavum vergae

2. They are present normally early in gestation but they close from back to front starting at 6 months gestation and are completely closed normally by 3-6 months after birth.

18.7 INFECTIVE CYSTIC LESIONS

Brain Abscess

* Well defined hypoechoic lesion with internal echoes and distal enhancement showing mass effect.

Subdural Effusion

* There is leakage of protein and fluid in subdural space due to inflammation of subdural veins
* Seen as crescentic extra-axial hypoechoic fluid collection in subdural space
* Usually resolve spontaneously
* Subdural effusion has to be differentiated from prominent subarachnoid spaces seen in atrophy and benign intracranial collection of infancy.

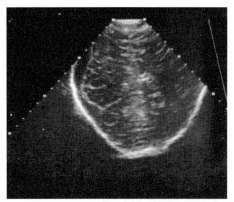

Fig. 18.7.1: Subdural effusion—small amount of fluid
is seen in the right subdural space

Subdural Effusion	Prominent Subarachnoid Spaces (Atrophy, Benign Extraxial Collection of Infancy)
Extraxial fluid does not extend between the cortical sulci	Extraxial fluid extends into the sulci
Cortical veins are displaced away from the inner table of the calvarium	Cortical veins course through the fluid and lie adjacent to the inner table of calvarium
Mass effect may be present	No mass effect
May be asymmetrical.	Usually symmetrical, if benign extracranial collection of infancy.

Benign Extra-axial Collection of Infancy

• Also known as benign enlargement of subarachnoid
  space in infancy and occurs due to delay in
  maturation of subarachnoid space

- Present between 2 to 6 months of age
- Microcephaly with no clinical signs of raised intracranial pressure
- CSF spaces are disproportionately larger with only mild prominence of ventricles. Subarachnoid spaces are more prominent in frontoparietal regions and are seen as widened cortical sulci, fissures and anterior interhemispheric fissure.

Empyema

- Seen as crescentic or lentiform extra-axial fluid collection with internal echoes usually in region of cerebral convexities and interhemispheric fissure on sonography with mass effect on the adjacent brain parenchyma.

18.8 VASCULAR LESIONS

Vein of Galen Malformation

- Aneurysmal dilatation of vein of Galen is the most common pathology of vascular causes
- Newborn usually presents with CHF
- USG shows a sonolucent mass posterior to 3rd ventricle causing obstructive hydrocephalus
- Color Doppler demonstrates turbulent bi-directional flow within the enlarged vein of Galen.

Varix of Vein of Galen

- Presents in young infants as cardiac failure
- US reveal a midline cystic structure above quadrigeminal plate
- Enlarged straight sinus.

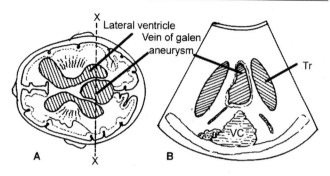

Fig. 18.8.1: A. Aneurysm of the vein of Galen. Axial (A) and posterior coronal (B) views. An aneurysm of the veiw of Galen is usually associated with lateral ventricular dilatation. The posterior coronal view was performed along line X-X

AV Malformation

- This congenital condition is rarely seen in infancy.
- Clinical presentation is with seizures and neurological deficit.
- Commonly supratentorial in location.
- Mostly solitary but may be multifocal in Wyburn-Mason and Rendu-Osler-Weber syndrome.
- Seen as multiple dilated tortuous vascular channels with arterial and venous signature on pulsed and color Doppler. Adjacent brain may show focal atrophy. Associated hemorrhage has variable appearance on US depending upon its stage. Formation of flow related aneurysms appear as focally dilated vascular channels in the feeding vessels or intranidal vessels.

18.9 TRAUMATIC CYSTIC LESIONS

Leptomeningeal Cyst
(Growing Fracture/Post-traumatic Cyst)

- Occurs as late complication of skull fracture with dural tear
- It is seen as an extra-axial, well defined, cystic structure with adjacent focal brain atrophy. It herniates through the bone defect into the subgaleal tissues.

Chronic Hematoma (Extra-axial)

- It appears as a cystic, well defined collection (crescentic – subdural, lenticular—epidural) in late stages of the hematoma due to clot lysis
- Extra-axial collection must be near 1 cm thick to be detected on sonography due to the near field artefact of 1 cm with most transducers.

18.10 INTRACRANIAL HEMORRHAGE

- Cerebral hemorrhage is a common CNS pathology in premature neonates due to presence of germinal matrix which involutes by 34 to 36 wk of gestation.

Germinal Matrix Hemorrhage

- Germinal matrix is a region of very thin walled veins and actively proliferating cells located in the subependymal layer of lateral ventricle

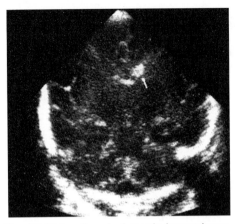

Fig. 18.10.1: Germinal matrix hemorrhage originating in germinal eminence

- Infants at greatest risk are those at gestational ages <30 weeks, of birth weight <1500 gm.

Causes

Prematurity with
- Hypoxia
- Hypertension
- Hypercapnia
- Hypernatremia
- Pneumothorax
- Rapid volume increase.

Germinal matrix hemorrhage may extend to
- Subependymal
- Intraventricular
  Intraparenchymal regions and is accordingly graded
as follows:

Grade I   : Subependymal hemorrhage

Grade II : Intraventricular extension without hydrocephalus

Grade III : Intraventricular hemorrhage with hydrocephalus

Grade IV : Intraparenchymal hemorrhage with or without hydrocephalus.

- Imaging
  — Echogenic focus in the region of caudate nucleus or caudothalamic groove.

Subependymal Hemorrhage

- *Imaging*
1. Echogenic clot in subependymal space, which may cause focal enlargement of choroid in caudothalamic groove.
2. As clot ages, it becomes less echogenic with center becoming hypoechoic.

Sequelae of Subependymal Hemorrhage

- May resolve completely
- Subependymal cyst
- Parenchymal/intraventricular extension leading to porencephaly/hydrocephalus respectively.

Intraventricular Hemorrhage without Hydrocephalus

1. Hyperechoic material that fills a portion of ventricular system.
2. Clot forms a cast of ventricle may obscure the ventricle due to complete filling of the lumen.

3. Thick echogenic choroid plexus.
4. Later echolucent center.
5. Low level echoes floating in a ventricle.
6. CSF-blood fluid levels.

Imaging after Development of Hydrocephalus

1. As ventricles dilate, clot and choroid plexus become better defined.
2. Echogenic clot adherent to the ventricular wall.
3. Clot movement may be seen with change in head position if clot is free.
4. Chemical ventriculitis due to presence of blood in CSF is seen as thickening of subependymal lining of ventricle.

Intraparenchymal Hemorrhage

• Most common sites are frontal and parietal lobes
• It is usually due to periventricular hemorrhagic venous infarction

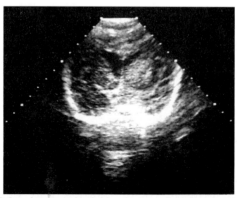

Fig. 18.10.2: Intracerebral bleed—a well defined echogenic lesion seen in the caudate region causing mass effect on frontal horn

— Large subependymal hemorrhage
— Compresses subependymal veins
— Hemorrhagic venous infarcts
— Intraparenchymal damage
— Later—porencephaly

- *Imaging*

1. Homogeneously echogenic mass extending into brain parenchyma usually associated with intraventricular hemorrhage.

2. As clot retracts, rim becomes echogenic with sonolucent center.

3. After 2-3 months of injury encephalomalacia or porencephalic cyst is formed.

18.11 ASPHYXIA

Birth asphyxia or perinatal hypoxia leads to:

1. Hemorrhage (intraparenchymal or subarachnoid). Imaging features of SAH
   - Enlarged Sylvian and interhemispheric fissure
   - Thickened sulci
   - Increased echogenicity within the sulci.

2. Periventricular leukomalacia (<34 week gestation)
   - It occurs in the watershed zone of periventricular area. These are B/L symmetrical lesions mainly around trigone but also extending to frontal lobes
   - On US, periventricular areas of increased echogenicity is the first visible change
   - On follow up, echogenicity may subside or may be replaced by cavitations
   - After several weeks, cyst collapse and disappear with reduction of periventricular white matter, deep cortical sulci and ventricular dilatation.

3. Ischemia (> 34 weeks gestation)

   Imaging features of infarction:
   - Arterial territorial distribution of injury
   - Echogenic parenchyma with mass effect from edema
   - Decreased sulcal definition
   - Lack of arterial pulsation at real-time examination
   - Lack of a vascular waveform and flow on pulsed Doppler and color Doppler respectively
   - Increased pulsation in the periphery of the infarcted with early collateral arterial vasculature.

Focal	*Diffuse*
Subcortical leukomalacia On USG, focal hypoechoic area is seen	Diffuse encephalomalacia Diffusely bright brain on USG There may be echogenic thalami in severe cases

18.12 SOLID INFECTIVE LESIONS

Cerebritis is the Focal or Diffuse Swelling with Mass Effect

- Focal cerebritis is seen as an echogenic area with mass effect in the cortex
- It leads to abscess formation in later stages.

Cerebral Edema

Imaging Features

- Diffusely echogenic brain parenchyma
- Poorly defined sulci

- Slit like ventricles
  The cause can be enumerated as:
1. Hypoxic-ischemic and other encephalopathy.
2. Meningo-encephalitis.
3. Trauma.

18.13 TUMORS

- Common neoplasms in this age group are:
  — astrocytoma (optic chiasm and hypothalamus),
  — choroid plexus papilloma,
  — primitive neuroectodermal tumors (PNET) and
  — ependymoma.
- Most CNS neoplasms are rare in infants
- If present, mostly supratentorial
- On US, they appear as highly reflective lesion with a mixed echopattern
- Mass effect and hydrocephalus are usually present.

18.14 CONGENITAL INTRACRANIAL INFECTION OF INFANT AND CHILDREN

TORCH organisms are most common cause of congenital CNS infections.

	CMV	*Toxoplasmosis*
Incidence	Most common	Second most common
Sites affected	Periventricular germinal matrix Cerebellum Brainstem Spinal cord	Basal ganglia Periventricular white matter Cortex

Contd...

Contd...

	CMV	*Toxoplasmosis*
Clinical features	Hepatosplenomegaly Jaundice Chorioretinitis Seizures Optic atrophy Hearing loss Mental retardation	Seizures Microcephaly
Calcifications	Periventricular	Scattered in basal ganglia and cortex
Ventricles	Enlarged due to atrophy	Hydrocephalus due to aqueductal stenosis
Migration anomalies	Present	Absent
Cerebral atrophy	Present	Not a feature

Rubella

- Incidence decreasing due to immunization
- Clinical features
    — Cataract, glaucoma, chorioretinitis
    — Microphthalmia
    — Cardiac malformations
    — Microcephaly
    — Deafness
- USG
1. Echogenic calcifications in basal ganglia and cortex with microcephaly.
2. Subependymal cysts in basal ganglia.

Herpes Simplex

- Neonatal herpes is HSV II

	HSV II (Genital herpes)	HSV I
Site of involvement	Usually responsible for neonatal infection Diffuse brain involvement	Usually affects adults Predilection for limbic system (Temporal lobe Cingulate gyrus)

- Imaging in HSV II:
1. Cystic encephalomalacia of periventricular white matter.
2. Hemorrhagic infarctions.
3. Scattered parenchymal calcification
4. Relative sparing of lower neuronal axis of thalamus, basal ganglia, cerebellum, brainstem.
5. *In utero* infection leads to:
   — Microcephaly
   — Intracranial calcification
   — Retinal dysplasias.

18.15 MENINGITIS

Infecting agents are:
1. Neonates: Group B *Streptococcus, E. coli, Listeria*
2. Infants: *H. influenzae*
   - Imaging

USG—In Acute Stage

1. Increased echogenicities in basal cisterns inter-hemispheric tissue and cortical sulci.

2. Lateral and 3rd ventricles are symmetrically compressed and subarachnoid spaces are effaced (due to diffuse brain edema).
3. Focal echogenic areas representing edema may be seen.
4. USG may be normal in uncomplicated cases.

Complications

1. Hydrocephalus.
2. Ventriculitis.

USG Shows

   a. Hydrocephalus.
   b. Echogenic debris within ventricle.
   c. Echogenic shaggy ependymal lining.
   d. Fibrous septae in ventricles that can cause trapped ventricle.
3. Subdural Effusion.
4. Empyema.

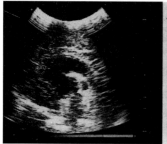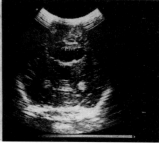

Figs 18.15.1A and B: Postmeningitis hydrocephalus lateral and third ventricles appear dilated, 4th ventricle is normal

5. Cerebritis and abscess.
6. Cerebrovascular complications, e.g. cerebral infarction, venous infarct, dural sinus thrombosis, mycotic aneurysm.

18.16 ENLARGED CHOROID PLEXUS

- Adherent clot (intraventricular hemorrhage)—serial scaaning may reveal complete resolution of the clot with or without development of hydrocephalus
- Infection (ventriculitis and choroid plexitis)
- Choroid plexus tumor (CPP)
    — Commonest site for CPP is lateral ventricle
    — Papilloma is well-defined lobulated masses causing enlargement of ventricular system.

19

Neonatal and Infant Spine

Complete visualization of spinal cord is possible in infant (due to presence of incompletely ossified vertebral arches) or in a child with a congenital or surgical bony defect. Various pathological conditions can be evaluated as:

1. Spinal dysraphism.
2. Postoperatives spine.
3. Spinal trauma.
4. Vascular.*
5. Tumors.

(*NB:Vascular anomalies do not usually present during infancy. However, if present, US reveal the anomaly and color Doppler helps in the hemodynamic assessment of the lesion).

19.1 SPINAL DYSRAPHISM

Overt Spinal Dysraphism

Non-skin Covered Back Mass (Spina Bifida Aperta)

1. Myelomeningocele.
2. Myelocele.

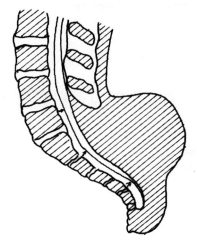

Fig. 19.1.1: A lumbosacral spine (sagittal) lipomyelomeningocele. Note the large defects in the neural arches of the lumbosacral vertebrae with a skin-covered herniated sac that is composed of fat contiguous with the subcutaneous fat that is growing into the dorsal aspect of the low-lying tethered spinal cord (arrows)

Skin Covered Black Mass (Spina Bifida Cystica)

1. Lipomyelomeningocele.
2. Myelocystocele.
3. Posterior meningocele.

Occult Spinal Dysraphism

1. Diastematomyelia.
2. Dorsal dermal sinus.
3. Spinal lipoma.
4. Tight filum terminale.
5. Anterior sacral meningocele.

6. Lateral thoracic meningocele.
7. Hydromyelia.
8. Split notochord syndrome.
9. Caudal regression syndrome.

19.2 SPINA BIFIDA APERTA

Myelomeningocele

- Most common congenital anomaly of central nervous system
- Occurrence 2 per 1000 live births

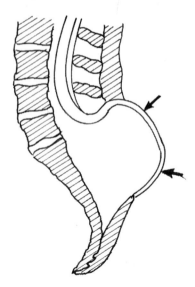

Fig. 19.2.1: Sagittal view of myelomeningocele at the level of the lumbosacral region with large defect in the neural arches of the lumbosacral verterae that has a herniated sac of exposed neural tissue (arrows) posteriorly and CSF anteriorly

- 98 percent have hydrocephalus.

Associated anomalies of brain are present—Chiari II malformation hydromyelia, arachnoid cyst, diastematomyelia.

In myelomeningocele the exposed part of the neural tissue (placode) is pushed above the surface of the back by the distended ventral subarachnoid space through the defect in the posterior arches of the spine soft tissues and dura.

US clearly distinguishes meningocele from myelomeningocele by demonstrating the presence of neural tissue in the protruding sac.

Myelocele

Has the more appearance as myelomeningocele but the herniated sac is flush with the plane of the back.

19.3 SPINA BIFIDA CYSTICA

Lipomyelomeningocele

Present as skin covered lumpy back masses. US reveals the subarachnoid space and cord bulging through the spina bifida into the subcutaneous tissues. The spinal canal is widened at the level of the defect. Common locations are lumbosacral, lumbar and lumbothoracic regions.

Myelocystocele

- Most common location is lumbosacral region
- Associations—cloacal exstrophy, partial sacral agenesis, hydromyelia

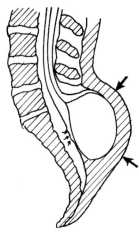

Fig. 19.3.1: Sagittal diagram of myelocystocele at the lumbo-sacral region in which a large dysraphic defect within the bone and a skin-covered back mass (the herniated sac) that contains the low-lying caudally splayed (small black arrows) spinal cord with a cyst (small white arrows) terminally are present. The subcutaneous fat (large black arrows) of the back is separated from the cyst by a tissue plane

US reveals—The herniated sac consists of the dilated central canal of the distal end of the low lying and tethered spinal cord, CSF and meninges.

The subcutaneous fat is clearly separated from the sac by a tissue plane.

Simple Posterior Meningocele

This is a skin covered back mass consisting of herniated sac of meninges (dura and arachnoid) with CSF protruding through a posterior bony defect in the spine. Most commonly formed in lumbosacral region. The

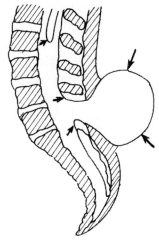

Fig. 19.3.2: Sagittal view of posterior meningocele herniation of a CSF sac (large black arrows) through a spina bifida at 1.5 (small black arrows). The conus is in the normal location (open arrows)

bony defect may involve the anterior aspect or lateral aspect resulting into anterior sacral and lateral thoracic meningoceles respectively and are classified under occult spinal dysraphism.

19.4 OCCULT SPINAL DYSRAPHISM

Diastematomyelia

- Complete or partial sagittal clefting of the spinal cord. The two hemicords typically reunite below the cleft
- More frequent in girls and common location is D9 to S1

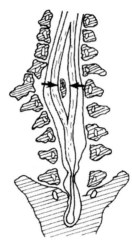

Fig. 19.4.1: Diagram (anteroposterior) of diastematomyelia with the area of clefting of the spinal cord (large black arrows), bony spur (small black arrow), and thickened filum

- Associated findings—segmentation anomalies of vertebral bodies
- US findings include clefting of spinal cord, spur (bony, fibrous, cartilaginous), hydromyelia (50%), fatty filum terminale, intradural lipoma and conus is low lying below L_2 level. These findings are demonstrated well on US
- 50 percent asymptomatic—this form of diastematomyelia does not have a spur and no duplication of meninges is seen.

Dorsal Dermal Sinus

- Epithelial tract that extends to a variable length from skin surface anteriorly and downwards into the associated soft tissue of the back. On US, it is seen as a linear or curvilinear echogenic tract reaching the spinal canal.

Spinal Lipomas

- Lipomyelocele
- Leptomyelolipoma
  Another form of spinal lipoma is lipomyelo-meningocele which is an overt spinal dysraphism
- Lipomas are lumps of subcutaneous soft tissues (connective tissue and fat) covered by skin and found most commonly in the lumbosacral region
- They may be associated with dermal sinuses, hemangiomas, nevi and hairy tufts
- Extension of the lesion is variable into the spinal canal through the defect in the midline dura, bone, muscle and fascia.

Lipomyelocele

Cord is intracanalicular and meninges do not bulge into the soft tissues.

On US, the echogenic lipoma is attached to the cord tethering the cord which is low and eccentric in position.

The lipoma may be limited to the filum or dura or extend into the central cord or along the cord.

Leptomyelolipoma

A term used when the lipoma has a large area of direct interface with the spinal cord.

This is a form of occult spinal dysraphism.

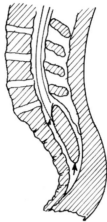

Fig. 19.4.2: Intradural lipoma (large black arrow) tethering a low-lying spinal cord (small black arrow), which is separated from the subcutaneous fat of the back by an obvious tissue plane (white arrows)

Intradural Lipoma

Intraspinal lipoma lie adjacent to the dorsal aspect of spinal cord. A tissue plane separates it from the adjacent subcutaneous fat of the back. Associated findings are spina bifida and a tethered cord.

Tight Filum Terminale

- On US, it appear as a thickened filum terminal > 2 mm in thickness
- Associated findings—spina bifida (50-70%) cases, low lying tethered cord (50%)

Anterior Sacral Meningocele

Defect anteriorly in sacrum with herniation of meninges and CSF into the presacral or pelvic area.

It may be associated with an anterior sacral teratoma.

Lateral Thoracic Meningocele

Sac protruding laterally into posterior mediastinum through intervertebral foramen or a lateral defect.

Commonly seen in patients with neurofibromatosis type I.

Hydromyelia

- Dilatation of central canal
- It may be focal, localized, multiple or diffuse
- It usually seen in association of other dysraphic states.
  US reveals the dilated central canal as separation of the normal echogenic line by an anechoic space.

Split Notochord

- Abnormal splitting or deviation of notochord covered by persistent partial or complete connection between any part of gut with spine, cord and or skin of back. Connection may be a tract, diverticulum, cyst, fistula or sinus.
  Presentation may be with a mass in chest, posterior mediastinum, spinal cord or as abdomen.
- Most common abnormality is mediastinal, dorsal enteric cyst presenting in childhood with respiratory symptoms (dyspnea, cyanosis), pulmonary infection and posterior mediastinal mass.

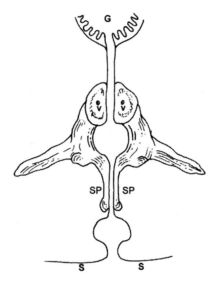

Fig. 19.4.3: Axial view of the split notochord syndrome: A tract extending from the gut (G) produces a sagittal cleft in the vertebral body (V) and spinous process (SP) to the skin (S) surface of the back

Caudal Regression Syndrome

- Characterised by absence of portions of the lower bony spine and spinal cord
- Associated findings are renal aplasia/dysplasia, neurogenic bladder, malformed external genitalia, and atresia and sirenomelia; club foot
- On US, conus ends abnormally high in spinal canal. Segmentation anomalies of vertebra and spina bifida are also seen.

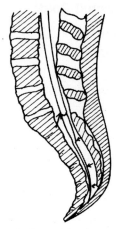

Fig. 19.5.1: Sagittal view of lumbosacral region. Conus (large black arrow) of the spinal cord, which is low-lying and tethered by a thickened fatty filum terminate (small black arrows) is detailed

19.5 TETHERED CORD

- Is a pathologically fixed spinal cord in an abnormal caudal location
- Child may be asymptomatic at birth but develops progressive neurological deficit with growth of the child.

Causes of Tethered Cord

- Lipomeningocele
- Intraspinal lipoma
- Thick filum terminale
- Dermal sinus

Risk Factors for Tethered Cord

- Atypical sacral dimples
- Subcutaneous lipomas
- Skin defect
- Hair tufts
- Skin tag
- Hemangioma
- Pigmented nevi
- Occult spinal dysraphism
- Dermal sinus
- Anorectal malformation
- Lipomeningocele
- Leptomyelolipoma
- Lipomyeloschisis.

Findings on US

- Level of conus below L_3
- Position of conus—eccentric especially dorsal
- Decreased cord oscillations (except in 1st 2 months).

19.6 SPINAL TRAUMA

Etiology

- Birth trauma
- Severely shaken infant
- Mechanism—longitudinal stretching of cord (hyper-extension of head) and rotational forces (forceps application)
  — Parts affected
  — Brainstem — (severely shaken infant)

— upper cervical cord – (cephalic delivery)
— lower cervical cord and upper thoracic segments (breech delivery).

Mode of Injury

— Cord laceration
— Transection
— Vascular injury at water shed areas.

US Features

Acute stage
• Cord discontinuity
• Cord swelling
• Abnormal reflectivity in swollen cord with non-visualisation of central canal
• Extra-axial hemorrhage within spinal cord, cisterna magna, soft tissues.

Chronic stage
• Cord atrophy—heterogeneous appearance and cysts.

19.7 TUMORS

• Spinal childhood tumors are rare especially during infancy
• Presentation—often nonspecific and non-neurological, motor weakness, spinal deformity cutaneous markers-dermoid, lipoma
  US findings depends upon the location of tumor:
• Extradural-displacement of dura inwards away from margins of spinal canal

- Intramedullary-discrete, diffuse heterogeneous area in a uniformly echopoor cord.
  — Cord expansion is present
- Extramedullary and intradural—the lesion compresses and displaces the cord and widens the subarachnoid space.

Extradural Tumors

US findings—expansion, disruption of vertebral body, dumbbell tumor with extension of paravertebral lesion into the canal that may be expanded due to tumor. Tumor appears to be of mixed echogenicity with areas of calcification.

Sacrococcygeal Tumors

- Rare congenital tumors (80% are benign, occurring more commonly in females)
- Association—anorectal malformation, anomalies of genitourinary tract, sacral vertebral anomaly
- Commonly occur as purely dorsal lesion or have a presacral mass as well.

US Reveals

- heterogeneous mass with calcification and spinal cord expansion
- displacement or encasement the spinal roots
- sacral erosion.

20

Gynecology and Obstetrics

20.1 FREE FLUID IN CUL-DE-SAC

1. Normal ovulation.
2. Follicular rupture.
3. Ruptured ectopic pregnancy or hemorrhagic cyst.
4. Generalized ascites.
5. Pelvic inflammatory diseases.
6. Following culdocentesis.
7. Pelvic abscess or hematoma.

The posterior cul-de-sac is the most posterior and inferior most reflection of the peritoneal cavity.

Normal Findings

In asymptomatic woman and can be seen during all phases of menstrual cycle.

Possible sources are—

- Blood or fluid caused by follicular rupture
- Blood caused by retrograde menstruation
- Increased capillary permeability of the ovarian surface caused by the influence of estrogen.

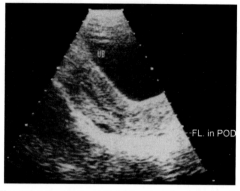

Fig. 20.1.1: Minimal fluid is seen in the pouch of Douglas following follicular rupture

Pathological Fluid Collection

Ruptured Ectopic Pregnancy

• Sonographic signs
• Live embryo in the adnexal
• Empty uterus
• Pseudogestational sac of ectopic pregnancy
• Particulate ascites
• Adnexal mass—rounded and complex
• Ectopic tubal ring
• Color Doppler imaging shows characteristic fire ring appearance.

Pelvic Inflammatory Disease

• Shows particulate fluid in the cul-de-sac
• Other findings of PID
• Endometritis—endometrial thickening or fluid, air if present, is diagnostic of endometritis

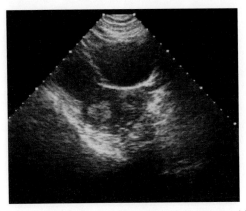

Fig. 20.1.2: Hyperplastic endometrium in uterus with cystic lesion in left ovary—ectopic pregnancy cannot be ruled out in such case

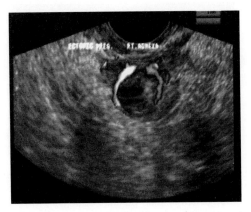

Fig. 20.1.3: Ectopic pregnancy—on color Doppler "ring of fire" appearance is seen

- Periovarian inflammation—enlarged ovaries with multiple cysts and indistinct margins. Pyosalpinx

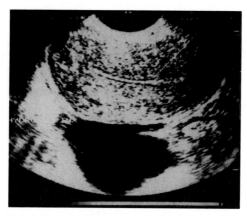

Fig. 20.1.4: Longitudinal scan shows markedly dilated fluid filled right fallopian tube

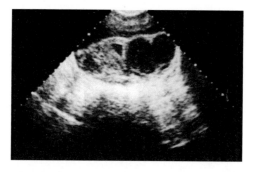

Fig. 20.1.5: Oblique scan showing, markedly dilated and thickened left fallopian tube filled with fluid with internal echoes. The endometrial cavity also contain fluid

    or hydrosalpinx—fluid filled fallopian tubes with or without internal echoes
* Tubo-ovarian complex

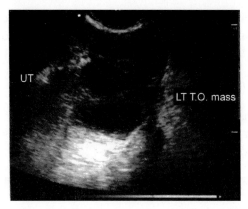

Fig. 20.1.6: Multiseptated complex heterogenous tubo-ovarian mass is seen in transverse section

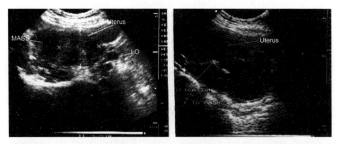

Fig. 20.1.7: Tubercular tubo-ovarian mass—longitudinal and transverse scan of pelvis showing normal left ovary and a complex adnexal mass on right side with heterogenous echotexture. The mass blends with posterior uterine wall. Also evidence of calcification is seen in mass

- Tubo-ovarian abscess—complex multiloculated mass with variable septations, irregular margins, and scattered internal echoes and debris-fluid level

- Pelvic abscess or hematoma—can occur in cul-de-sac and sonographic appearance is similar to these conditions elsewhere in the body.

Generalized Ascites

The posterior cul-de-sac is a potential space and because of its location it is the frequently initial site for intraperitoneal fluid collection.

20.2 CYSTIC PELVIC MASSES

1. Obstructed uterus.
2. Cystic adnexal masses.
3. Extra-adnexal cystic masses.

Obstructed Uterus

Obstructed genital tract results in collection of blood and/or reactions in the uterus and/or vagina. Before menstruation hydrometrocolpos while after menstruation hematometrocolpos results from various causes like- *imperforate hymen, vaginal atresia/stenosis or blocked rudimentary uterine horn. Endometrial or cervical tumors, postradiation fibrosis* may also result in hemato/hydrometra.

Before puberty, US reveals anechoic collection within the genital tract, while hemorrhage and infection result in echoes, echogenic material or fluid-fluid level within the collection.

Cystic Adnexal Masses

Include both non-neoplastic and neoplastic lesions.

Non-neoplastic Lesions

- Functional cysts—include follicular, corpus luteal, hemorrhagic
- Endometriosis and theca lutein cysts
- Paraovarian (paratubal) cysts
- Tubal lesions as hydro/pyosalpinx.

Functional cysts are the most common cause of ovarian enlargement in young woman. Most functional cysts usually resolve within one or two menstrual cycle and follow up is usually not required for small simple cysts.

However, follow up is usually required in larger or hemorrhagic cysts at a different phase of menstrual cycle usually in 6 weeks.

Neoplastic lesions like serous and mucinous variety of ovarian cystadenoma can present as simple cystic mass in adnexal region. One or two thin septa may be present in it. Mucinous variety also shows low level echos in the cysts.

Extra-adnexal Cystic Mass

- Peritoneal inclusion cysts
- Mesenteric cyst
- Urinoma
- Lymphocele
- Hematoma
- Bladder diverticulum, dilated distal ureters
- Ectopic gestation
- Fluid distended bowel
- Loculated pelvic abscess.

Peritoneal inclusion cyst—on sonography peritoneal inclusion cyst appears as multiloculated cystic masses. The diagnostic finding is presence of an intact ovary amid septations and fluid. This indicates an extra ovarian origin of the mass. The ovary may be located centrally or displaced peripherally.

Mesenteric or Omental Cysts

Mesenteric cyst usually found in root of mesentery, omental cyst usually seen adjacent to the bowel.

Sonographically they appear as unilocular cystic mass that may be septated. Rarely a fat-fluid level may be seen. Differentiation from other cystic lesion may be difficult.

Lymphocele—disruption of lymphatic vessels following surgery or trauma results in the development of lymphocele.

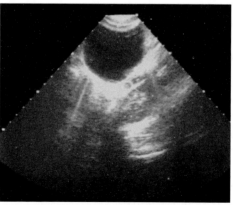

Fig. 20.2.1: Mesenteric cyst—a large cystic anechoic SOL with thin wall seen displacing the bowel loops

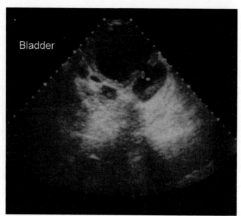

Fig. 20.2.2: Narrow neck diverticulum as seen from the posterior wall of urinary bladder with evidence of debris inside

Most commonly seen in pelvis, in the abdominal peritoneal recesses or in the retroperitonium.

Uncomplicated lymphocele appears as echo poor collection mimicking loculated ascites or mesenteric cyst. Septation or floating debris seen when they are complicated by hemorrhage or infection.

Bladder Diverticulum

Most result from bladder outlet obstruction. Bladder mucosae herniate through weak areas in the wall.

On sonography cystic lesion seen to communicate with the UB. Internal echogenicity varies depending on the diverticulum contents.

Fluid Distended Bowel

Can mimic adnexal mass but continuation with bowel loop may help in identification. Presence of peristalsis also confirms bowel.

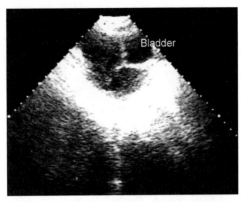

Fig. 20.2.3: Pelvic abscess—collection seen adjacent to bladder with debris inside it. It was a postoperative case of acute appendicitis

Loculated Pelvic Abscess

Appendiceal, diverticular and postoperative abscess. Appears as fluid collections having echoes, ± septa and well defined irregular wall. Presence of air appears as highly reflective foci with reverberation artefacts and is specific of an abscess.

20.3 COMPLEX PELVIC MASS

- Uterine lesions—complex uterine collection, large necrotic tumors like fibroids, leiomyosarcoma
- Ovarian lesions
  - Hemorrhagic cyst
  - Endometrioma
  - Ectopic pregnancy
  - Tubo-ovarian abscess

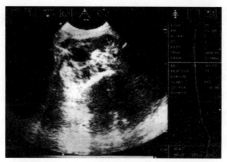

Fig. 20.3.1: Tubo-ovarian abscess

— Tumors like teratoma/dermoid, malignant tumors like cystadenoma and necrotic germ cell tumors.
- Extra-adnexal lesions like complex collections (abscess), hematoma, loculated ascites, complex bowel masses, necrotic soft tissue tumors, etc.

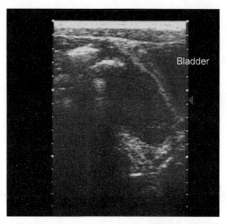

Fig. 20.3.2: Pelvic hematoma—in this case of blunt abdominal trauma. A collection is seen in the pelvis with internal echoes inside it

20.4 SOLID PELVIC MASSES

Uterine (usually midline)
- Fibroids
- Adenomyosis
- Endometrial hyperplasia
- Endometrial carcinoma

Cervical—fibroid, carcinoma

Off-midline
- Adnexal
  Ovarian
  — Non-neoplastic—ovarian torsion, oophoritis, polycystic ovary
  — Neoplastic—benign (fibroma, thecoma, Brenner tumor) and malignant (surface epithelial tumors—cystadenocarcinoma, endometroid carcinoma; germ cell tumors; sex chord tumors).
  Tubal
  — Fallopian tube carcinoma
  Broad ligament
  — Fibroid
- Non-adnexal
  — Bowel masses
  — Soft tissue tumors
  — Bladder masses
  — Nodal masses.

20.5 ADNEXAL MASSES

Cystic Ovarian Mass

  I. Completely cystic.

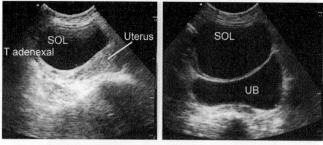

Fig. 20.5.1: Transverse and oblique view—a well defined anechoic cyst—serous cystadenoma

- Functional cyst—follicular cyst, corpus luteal cyst (uncomplicated)
- Endometrioma
- Hydrosalpinx
- Cyst adenoma
- Cystic teratoma
- Paraovarian cyst
- Serous/mucinous cystadenoma
- Serous/mucinous cystadenocarcinoma.

II. Multiple cysts—endometriomas.

III. Septated—cystadenomas, theca lutein cysts, massive edema of ovary.

Solid

- Ovarian tumors
- Ovarian torsion
- Oophoritis
- Polycystic ovaries
- Fallopian tube carcinoma.

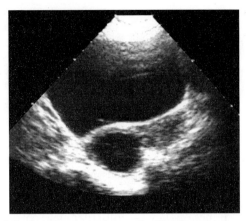

Fig. 20.5.2: Functional ovarian cyst with internal hemorrhage is seen as well-defined rounded lesion with internal echoes inside it

Follicular cysts are discovered incidentally on sonographic examination. They appear as unilocular, anechoic cyst more than 2.5 cm in diameter.

Corpus luteal cyst is less common but larger and more symptomatic than follicular cyst. They are more prone to rupture and hemorrhage like corpus lutein cysts hemorrhage cyst—clinically present with acute pelvic pain. On us they may appear as a cyst with internal echoes, complex cystic lesion with internal echoes and septae, fluid-fluid level within it or a hyperechoic lesion (in an acute, hemorrhagic cyst) mimicking a solid lesion.

Theca Lutein Cyst

There are associated with high levels of HCG (patients with trophoblastic disease, ovarian hyperstimulation

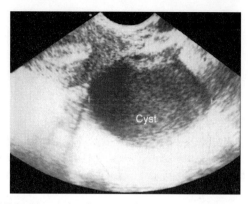

Fig. 20.5.3: Hemorrhagic cyst of ovary well-defined rounded hypoechoic cystic lesion with low level echoes and forming a level seen on the left of scan

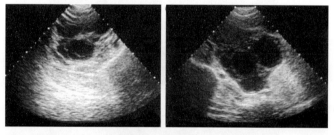

Fig. 20.5.4: Theca lutein cyst seen on follow-up case of hydatiform mole. Bilateral adnexal lesions are showing multiseptated appearance

syndrome). On US bilateral, multilocular large cysts are seen.

Endometrioma—defined as presence of functional endometrial tissue outside the uterus. Localized form is referred to as endometrioma or chocolate cyst.

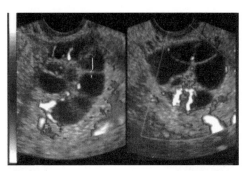

Fig. 20.5.5: Intraovarian perfusion seen in a case of ovarian stimulation

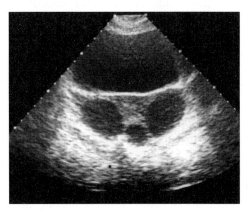

Fig. 20.5.6: Endometrioma

Diffuse form is usually asymptomatic and multiple and not evident on ultrasound.

In the localized form ultrasound reveals a unilocular or multilocular (due to satellite cysts) predominantly cystic mass containing diffuse homogenous low-level internal echoes. A fluid-fluid level may be seen. Bright reflectors may be seen in the wall. Endometrioma are commonly confused with hemorrhage cyst or tubo-ovarian abscesses. Significant decrease in size is noticed in hemorrhagic cyst unlike in endometrioma. Tubo-ovarian abscess present with acute pelvic pain associated with fever.

Dermoid Cyst

- Seen in young patients
- Completely anechoic form can also be seen.

Paraovarian or Paratubal Cyst

- 10 percent of all adnexal mass, mesothelial or paramesonephric in origin, most common in 3rd decade
- Unilocular cystic lesion in the broad ligament
- Frequently located superior to the uterine fundus
- Normal ipsilateral ovary.

Massive Edema of the Ovary

- Rare condition, resulting from partial or intermittent torsion of the ovary/causing venous or lymphatic but not arterial obstruction
- This results in ovarian enlargement d/t marked edema of ovarian stroma
- Sonography shows multicystic adnexal mass.

Hydrosalpinx

Fluid filled dilated fallopian tube seen in adnexal as a well defined walled tubular, ovoid with kinked configuration collection. *Pyosalpinx* demonstrates internal echoes as well.

Solid Masses: Ovarian tumors discussed later.

Ovarian Torsion

- Is an acute abdominal condition of childhood or adolescence. May occur in association with ovarian cysts and tumors m/c with teratomas
- Caused by partial or complete rotation of the ovarian pedicle on its axis
  Sonography shows
- Unilaterally enlarged ovary
- Multiple cortical follicles in an enlarged ovary-considered as specific sign but not always present
- Color Doppler shows absent flow from the affected ovary.

Polycystic Ovarian Disease (PCOD)

- This complex endocrinologic disorder results in chronic anovulation
- Bilateral enlarged spheroidal ovaries containing multiple small follicles and stromal hypertrophy and increased echogenicity
- The follicles measures from .5 to .8 cm in size with more than five in each ovary
- Follicles persist on serial studies as a string of pearls
- An elevated LH/FSH ratio is characteristic.

Carcinoma of Fallopian Tube

- Least common (<1%) of all gynecological malignancy

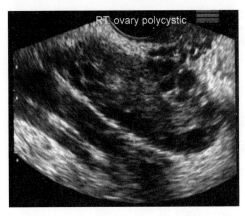

Fig. 20.5.7: PCOD: gray scale image showing an enlarged right ovary (volume: 28.78 ml) with small peripheral follicles and increased stromal echogenicity

- Most frequent in postmenopausal woman.
- Usually involves the distal end of the tube
- Present as sausage shaped solid or cystic mass with papillary projection.

20.6 OVARIAN TUMORS

Benign	*Malignant*
1. Cystic	1. Cystic
• Serous cystadenoma	• Serous cystadenocarcinoma
• Mucinous cyst adenoma	• Mucinous cystadeno-
• Teratoma/dermoid cyst	• Carcinoma endometroid

Contd...

Table contd...

2. Solid	2. Solid
Brenner	• Endometroid granulosa cell tumor. Dysgerminoma
Thecomas	Endodermal sinus tumor (yolk sac tumor)
Fibromas	Metastatic

BENIGN TUMORS

Cystadenoma

- Most common cystic ovarian tumor
- May be serous or mucinous
- Sonographically, appears as large thin walled unilocular cystic masses ± thin septations and papillary projections
- Multilocular lesion containing low level echoes in its dependant part suggests the mucinous variety.

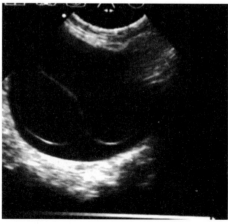

Fig. 20.6.1: Serous cystadenoma—large anechoic lesion with thin septae in right adnexal region

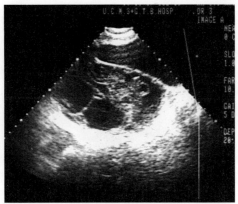

Fig. 20.6.2: Cystadenocarcinoma—large complex mass with cystic and solid areas and multiple septae in right adnexa

Cystic Teratoma

- Most common ovarian neoplasm seen in reproductive age group
- 10-20 percent are bilateral.

  Sonographic appearance is variable ranging from completely cystic appearance to erroneously interpreted solid lesion.

On US
- Unilocular anechoic/hypoechoic cyst with thick/thin walls
- Hyperechoic mural nodule may be present
- Focal/diffuse area of greatly increased echogenicity often with shadowing
- Demonstration of teeth, fat-fluid level, hair-fluid level is a specific sign
- Echogenic dermoid may be misinterpreted for bowel gas and missed completely.

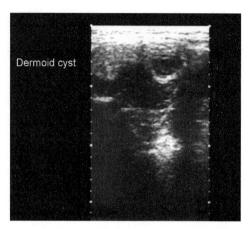

Fig. 20.6.3: Dermoid cyst—a complex mass lesion in right adnexa with solid and cystic areas. Multiple linear hyperechogenic interfaces floating in the mass

Solid Benign Ovarian Tumor

- Brenner tumor, Granulosa cell tumor, thecomas and fibroma are indistinguishable from each other and from pedunculated uterine fibroid
- Thecomas and granulosa cell tumor are estrogenically active
- On US, they appear as well defined, rounded, solid lesion causing attenuation of sound beam
- Left sided pleural effusion and ascites associated with fibroma is called Meig's syndrome.

MALIGNANT OVARIAN NEOPLASM

- Third most common gynecologic malignancy and has the highest mortality rate.

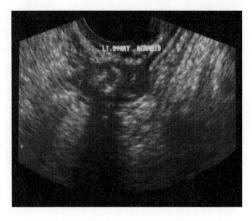

Fig. 20.6.4: Gray scale image showing an ovarian dermoid

US FEATURES OF MALIGNANT OVARIAN LESIONS

1. Solid mass.
2. Mass more than 10 cm (except thin walled unilocular cyst).
3. Thick septa (>3 mm).
4. Mural nodule.
5. Thick irregular solid mass.
6. Poorly defined margins.
7. Adherent bowel loops.
8. Ascites.
    I. Cystadenocarcinoma (serous and mucinous)
    - appear as multiloculated cystic masses having solid nodules and papillary excrescences
    - 8 percent are completely solid without cystic component.

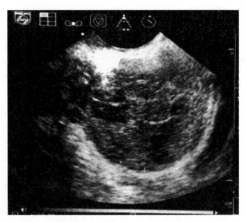

Fig. 20.6.5: Solid ovarian mass lesion suggestive of ovarian malignancy

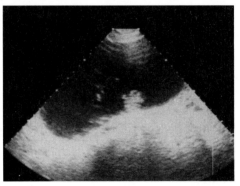

Fig. 20.6.6: Malignant ovarian mass—an irregular cystic lesion of right ovary with mural nodule and echogenic branching septae

II. Endometroid tumors
- These tumors have better prognosis as they are detected early. Thirty percent of patients have associated endometrial carcinoma.

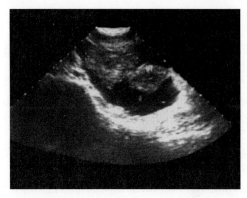

Fig. 20.6.7: Transverse scan of pelvis shows heterogenous, predominantly echogenic ovarian mass surrounded by free fluid

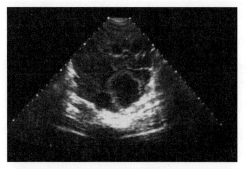

Fig. 20.6.8: Mucinous cystadenoma and cystadenocarcinoma of ovary

- US reveals
  - Cystic mass with papillary projections or predominantly solid mass with necrosis.
III. Malignant germ cell tumors {Dysgerminoma and endodermal sinus tumors}
  - Younger age group is affected

- α-fetoprotein is raised in endodermal sinus tumors.

  US reveals solid echogenic masses having small areas of necrosis.

IV. Metastatic tumor
- Metastasis to ovaries arises most commonly from gastric, colonic and breast malignancies
- Gastric and colonic metastases contain mucin secreting 'signet ring' cells and are called *Krukenberg tumors.*

  US shows bilateral solid lesion. A complex mass may be seen.

20.7 UTERINE MASSES

Benign

- Uterine fibroids (90%)
- Pyometra
- Hematohydrocolpos
- Transient uterine contraction (during pregnancy)
- Bicornuate uterus
- Adenomyosis
- Intrauterine pregnancy
- Lipoleiomyoma.

Malignant

- Cervical carcinoma
- Endometrial carcinoma
- Leiomyosarcoma
- Invasive trophoblastic disease.

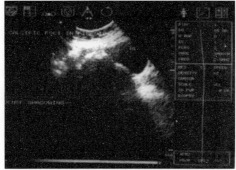

Fig. 20.7.1: Fibroid uterus

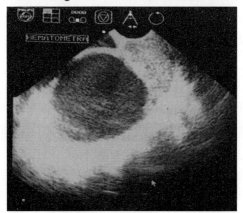

Fig. 20.7.2: Hematometrocolpos

Leiomyoma

Most common neoplasm of uterus and most common cause of enlargement of nonpregnant uterus.

Clinical Features

• Usually asymptomatic

- However, pain and uterine bleeding are usual presenting features.

Types
- Subserosal
- Intramural (most common)
- Submucosal (most symptomatic).

US
- Well defined hypoechoic lesion with sound beam attenuation
- Uterine contour deformity, displaced/distorted endometrial echo.

As they are estrogen dependent:
- During pregnancy, 50 percent increase in size, decrease in echogenicity due to degeneration and necrosis.

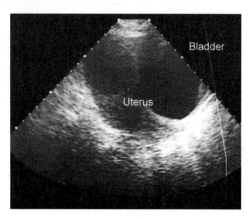

Fig. 20.7.3: Fibroid uterus—well-defined round hypoechoic solid lesion seen in the region of fundus

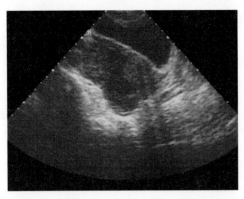

Fig. 20.7.4: Multiple uterine fibroids showing degeneration

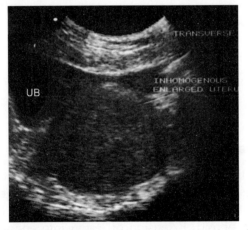

Fig. 20.7.5: Multiple fibroids—inhomogenously enlarged uterus with posterior lobulated margin in longitudinal section with multiple poorly resolved hypoechoic areas

- Postmenopausal regression in size and calcification occurs.

Focal Myometrial Contraction

This is a transient, focal contraction of the myometrium of pregnant uterus and commonly confused with an intramural fibroid.

On US, it appears similar in echotexture as the myometrium, no attenuation of sound beams is present. Disappears after some time.

Adenomyosis

Localized form of adenomyosis/adenomyomas appears as inhomogeneous circumscribed areas in the myometrium having indistinct margins and containing anechoic spaces.

Lipoleiomyoma

- Asymptomatic lesion
  US shows a highly echogenic attenuating mass within the myometrium.

Cervical Carcinoma

A condition diagnosed clinically. US reveals a solid retrovesical mass which is hypoechoic or heterogeneous in echotexture. The lesion is indistinguishable from a cervical fibroid. Extension of lesion into endometrial canal causes cervical stenosis and pyometra formation.

Leiomyosarcoma

- Only 1 percent of leiomyomas undergo sarcomatous change

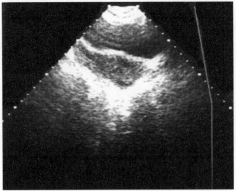

Fig. 20.7.6: Carcinoma cervix—longitudinal scan of the cervix shows an irregular growth. Base of the bladder is not involved

- Patients are usually asymptomatic or may present with uterine bleeding
- US shows a rapidly growing or degenerating leiomyoma with or without local invasion or distant metestasis.

Rudimentary Horn of Bicornuate Uterus

This congenital lesion may present as a mass lesion if it contains functional endometrium and then retention of menstrual blood can occur.

20.8 DIFFUSE UTERINE ENLARGEMENT

1. Diffuse leiomyomatosis
2. Adenomyosis
3. Endometrial carcinoma.

20.9 THICKENED ENDOMETRIUM

1. Early intrauterine pregnancy.
2. Incomplete abortion.

3. Ectopic pregnancy.
4. Retained products.
5. Trophoblastic disease.
6. Endometrial hyperplasia.

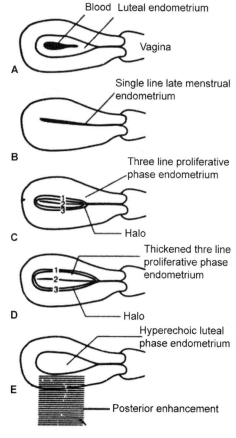

Fig. 20.9.1: Uterine endometrium in different phases of menstruation

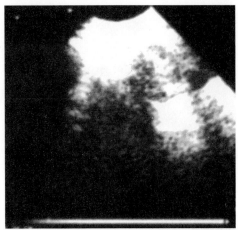

Fig. 20.9.2A: Incomplete abortion: thickened endometrium only, transabdominal scan showing uterus with thickened endometrium

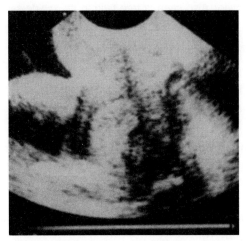

Fig. 20.9.2B: Incomplete abortion: thickened endometrium only, transvaginal scan showing the thickened endometrium more clearly

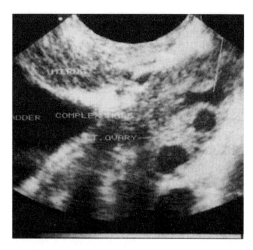

Fig. 20.9.3: Ecotopic pregnancy: adnexal mass—transvaginal scan reveals a complex mass in the (L) adnexa separate from the (L) ovary. Also seen is free fluid in the cul-de-sac

7. Endometrial polyp.
8. Endometrial cancer.
9. Endometritis.
10. Adhesions.
11. Foreign body (IUCD).

Sonographic appearance and thickness of endometrium varies 'with the phase of menstrual cycle.

Profilerative phase: Triple line endometrium—4-8 mm thick.

Secretory phase: Hyperechoic—7 to 14 mm, acoustic enhancement.

Postmenstrual: asymptomatic—upto 8 mm
Symptomatic (P/V bleeding)—up to 4 mm.

Early Intrauterine Pregnancy

Earliest detection on US is at 4 week 3 days by TVS, and 5 wk by TAS. The gestation sac is seen as a small collection surrounded by moderate level echoes of uniform thickness located eccentrically within the endometrium.

- hCG level double every 2 days in early intrauterine pregnancy.

Incomplete Abortion, Retained Products

An enlarged uterus with thickened endometrium with echogenic/heterogeneous material ± fluid in a proper clinical setting suggests the diagnosis.

Ectopic Pregnancy

- Clinical symptoms-missed period, P/V bleeding pain
- hCG-raised less than in normal pregnancy.

US Reveals

- Thick echogenic endometrium ± fluid collection (pseudogestational sac)
- Adnexal mass—cystic, complex ± live embryo, tubal ring on colour doppler imaging
  — Free fluid in POD.

Gestational Trophoblastic Disease

This is a proliferative disease of trophoblasts presenting as hydatiform mole (benign form) or as malignant forms—invasive mole or choriocarcinoma.

- Most common form is hydatiform mole.

Risk factors

- Women at end of their reproductive age group
- Previous similar history.

US Shows

Ist trimester mole
 — Simulates a blighted ovum
 — Threatened abortion
 — Small echogenic mass filling the uterine cavity.
IInd trimester mole
 — Large moderately echogenic mass filling the uterine cavity.
 — Cystic fluid containing spaces within it.
- Doppler—low impedance, high flow with high systolic and diastolic velocities
- β–hCG is raised more than in a normal pregnancy
- Complications—Hemorrhage seen as crescentic anechoic regions surrounding the tumor.

Theca Lutein Cysts

Variations of molar pregnancy
1. Coexistent mole and fetus
 • One normal fetus
 • Molar transformation of one binovular twin placenta.
2. Partial mole (triploidy)
 • Identifiable fetal tissue/fetus which is growth retarded or dystrophic
 • Formed placenta, which has numerous cystic spaces.

3. Invasive mole
   - Hydatidiform mole (villous pattern preserved) with local invasion
   - US—involvement of myometrium with or without extension into parametrium.
4. Choriocarcinoma—50 percent cases are preceded by molar pregnancy
   - No identifiable villous pattern seen while necrosis and hemorrhage are present.

US

   - Tumor extends into myometrium with or without parametrium
   - Metastasis to lung, brain liver, bone, GIT, skin.
5. Placental site trophoblastic tumor
   - paucity of syncytiotrophoblasts and therefore low levels of b HCG.
   - Levels of Human Placental Lactogen is increased
   - lack of chorionic villi, lack of necrosis and hemorrhage
   - US—no specific appearance.

Endometrial Hyperplasia

- Proliferation of glands leading to increased gland/stroma ratio
- Diffuse involvement
- With or without cellular atypia, 25 percent of hyperplasia with atypia progress to endometrial carcinoma
- Common cause of abnormal uterine bleeding developing from unapposed estrogen stimulation in post or perimenopausal women.

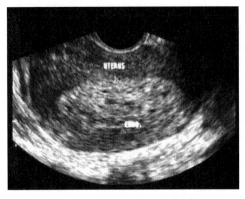

Fig. 20.9.4: Increased endometrial thickness in a case of endometrial hyperplasia

Causes

- Estrogen HRT
- Persistant anovulatory
- polycystic ovarian disease during reproductive age group
- Estrogen producing tumors-granulosa cell tumors and thecoma
- Tamoxifen effect.

US

- Reveals thickened echogenic endometrium having well defined margins
- Small cysts may be seen in cystic hyperplasia.

Endometrial Polyp

- Important condition presenting in peri- or post-menopausal females as uterine bleeding

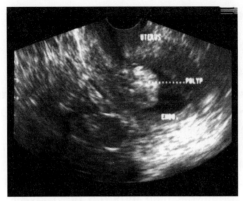

Fig. 20.9.5: Endometrial polyp seen as a localised echogenic lesion in the endometrium

- In younger females-They present as inter-menstrual bleeding or menometrorrhagia or infertility

US Reveals

- a nonspecific, echogenic, localized (central or eccentric) endometrial thickening with or without cysts
- Thickening may be diffuse
- On sonohysterography, it is seen as rounded, focal, echogenic mass within the endometrial cavity. Pedicle shows a feeding artery on color Doppler imaging.

It is easily differentiated from submucosal fibroids on sonohysterography which shows a rounded, hypoechoic sound attenuating lesion bulging into the endometrial cavity lined by normal thickness of endometrium.

Endometrial Carcinoma

- Presents as peri or postmenopausal bleeding.

US Reveals

- Thickened endometrium (>8 mm in asymptomatic or >4 mm in symptomatic postmenopausal females), mostly focal but can be diffuse
- Endometrium–echogenic/mixed echogenicity/hypoechoic
- Endometrial-myometrial interface-absence of subendometrial halo indicates deep invasion
- Cervical extension causes hemato- or pyometra
- it may appear as a heterogeneously, enlarged uterus with lobulations.

Endometritis

- Clinical presentation with features of pelvic inflammatory disease.

US

Prominent echogenic endometrium with or without fluid with debris, debris-fluid level presence of air is diagnostic.

Other features of PID like pyosalpinx (tubular shape cystic structure with folded configuration and echoes within it), complex tubo-ovarian masses, and fluid in POD.

Adhesions

- Clinical presentation is with h/o infertility, scanty menstruation

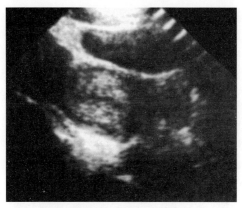

Fig. 20.9.6: Endometriosis

- History of D/C is present
- US—Irregular, echogenic, endometrium with areas of focal thickening
- Sonohysterography demonstrates the synechia
- Foreign body—IUCD.

Endometrial Fluid

- Normal finding
  - Menstruation
  - Postmenopausally (small amount)
- Endometritis
- Early pregnancy
- Ectopic gestation
- Obstructed uterus
  - Congenital conditions like imperforate hymen, vaginal septum, vaginal atresia, rudimentary horn of bicornuate uterus

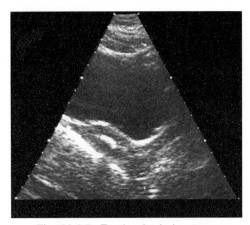

Fig. 20.9.7: Foreign body in uterus

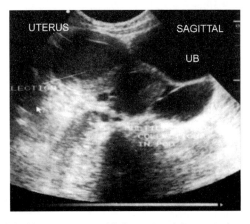

Fig. 20.9.8: Hematometra with hematosalpinx—uterine cavity is distended with fluid showing low level echoes. Dilated fallopian tube is showing low level echoes, septal and echogenic clot inside it

— Cervical stenosis
— Cervical carcinoma
— Endometrial carcinoma
— Post irradiation fibrosis.

Foreign Body (IUCD)

It is seen as a thick linear echo with a distal shadowing.

20.10 D/D OF THICKENED PLACENTA

Causes

1. Maternal diabetes.
2. Rhesus isoimmunization.
3. Fetal hydrops.
4. Triploidy.
5. Intrautuine infections.
6. Maternal severe anemia.
7. Fetal anemia.
8. Fetal hydrops.
9. Homozygous alpha-thalassemia.

Salient Features

- Placenta is called thickened when it measures > 4 cm in thickness at the cord incertion
- Most of the above causes are better evaluated by microscopic and biochemical eualuation of maternal blood
- Karyotyping is an essential step in evaluation
- USG has a corroborative role in evaluating structural abnormalities in above conditions, e.g. fetal hydrops chromosomal abnormalities.

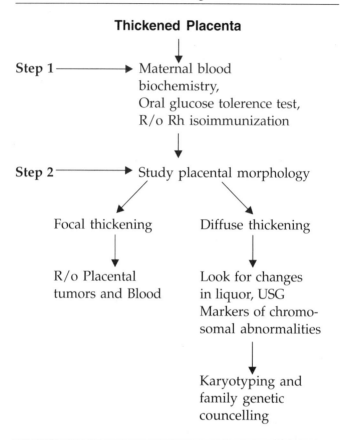

Thickened Placenta

Step 1 ⟶ Maternal blood biochemistry, Oral glucose tolerence test, R/o Rh isoimmunization

Step 2 ⟶ Study placental morphology

Focal thickening

R/o Placental tumors and Blood

Diffuse thickening

Look for changes in liquor, USG Markers of chromosomal abnormalities

Karyotyping and family genetic councelling

20.11 ULTRASOUND SIGNS OF CHROMOSOMAL ABNORMALITY

Generalized Signs
which are Important even if isolated

1. Borderline ventriculomegaly.
2. Posterior fossa abnormality.

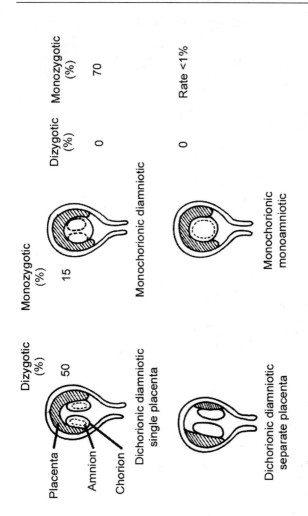

Fig. 20.11.1: Placenta and membranes in twin pregnancies

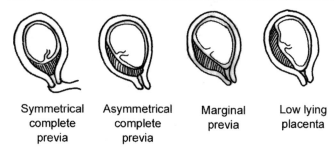

Fig. 20.11.2: Abnormalities of the placenta

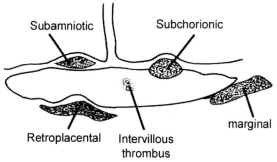

Fig. 20.11.3: Placental haemorrhage

3. Cystic hygroma.
4. Nuchal fold thickness.
5. Nuchal translucency.
6. Atrioventricular septal defects.
7. Double outlet right ventricle.
8. Omphalocele.
9. Duodenal atresia.
10. Echogenic bowel.
11. Genitourinary abnormality.
12. Non-immune hydrops.

Important Specific Signs

Trisomy 21

1. Cystic hygroma.
2. Non-immune hydrops.
3. Nuchal thickening.
4. Hydrothorax.
5. Gut atresias.
6. Protruding tongue.
7. Cleinodactyly.
8. Increased distance between 1st and 2nd toes.

Trisomy 18

1. IUGR.
2. Single umbilical artery.
3. Cystic hygroma.
4. Microcephaly/dolichocephaly.
5. Megacisterna magna.
6. Omphalocele.
7. Renal dysplasias.
8. Rocker bottom feet.

Trisomy 13

1. Cyclopia.
2. Anophthalmia.
3. Cleft lip/palate
4. Low set deformed ear.
5. Holoprosencephaly.
6. Duplicated kidney.
7. Polydactyly.
8. Rocker bottom feet.

Triploidy

1. Early onset IUGR.
2. Myelomeningocele.

3. Agenesis of corpus callosum.
4. Micrognathia.
5. Sloping forehead.
6. Post axial polydactyly/syndactyly.
7. Molar placenta.
8. Renal cortical cyst.

Turner's Syndrome

1. Cystic hygroma.
2. Non-immune hydrops.
3. Brachycephaly.
4. Small mandible.
5. Co-arctation of aorta.
6. Horse-shoe kidney.
7. Cubitus valgus.
8. Short-stature.

Approach to Mother having USG signs of chromosomal abnormality

↓

Fetal anomaly seen

↓

————————*Detailed USG evaluation*

↙   ↘

Isolated abnormality   **>1 abnormality**

↓   ↓

Consider Genetic/   Refer for Genetic
Obstetric Counseling   Counseling and
                         Fetal Karyotyping

→ Follow "Rule of Three"

↓

i.e. Head; Body; Extremities and thereby systematic evaluation of each part.

20.12 ABSENT PREGNANCY TEST WITH ABSENT I/U PREGNANCY

Causes

1. Ectopic pregnancy.
2. Very early I/U pregnancy.
3. Recent abortion.
4. Molar pregnancy/gestational trophoblastic neoplasia.

Salient Features

1. *Ectopic Pregnancy:*
   - *Specific Feature:* Live embryo in the adnexa.
   - *Nonspecific Feature* (Need β-hCG correlation)
     - Empty uterus.
     - Pseudogestational sac in uterus.
     - Particulate ascites.
     - Adnexal mass.
     - Ectopic tubal ring.
   - *Nonsupportive Features:*
     - Live intrauterine pregnancy.
     - Peritrophoblastic flow.
     - Intradecidual sign/double decidual sac sign.
   - Slow rising β-hCG, i.e. doubling time <2 days.
2. *Very Early Intrauterine Pregnancy*
   - Pregnancy test becomes positive at approximately 23 days. The earliest sonographic sign of pregnancy, i.e. Intradecidual sign is detected at approximately 25 days. During this window period of 2 days confusion may occur.

- It is always wise to screen after 72 hours in case of any confusion.
3. *Recent Abortion*
   In case of positive pregnancy test with USG showing no i/u pregnancy serial monitoring of β-hCG should be done. In cases of abortion a falling titer is seen in maternal serum.
4. *Gestational Trophoblastic Neoplasia*
   Uterus is enlarged with cavity filled with multiple small vesicles and soft-tissue nodules. Fetal parts and myometrial invasion may or may not be seen β-hCG levels are quite high.

20.13 FETAL CAUSES OF ABNORMALITIES IN LIQUOR VOLUME

Causes

A. *Oligohydramnios:*
   - Fetal demise /IUD
   - Renal/bladder abnormalities
     - PUV
     - Prune Belly syndrome
     - ARPCKD
     - BRA
   - IUGR
   - Post dated pregnancy.
B. *Polyhydramnios:*
   - Cardiovascular decompansation
   - Diaphragmatic hernia
   - Anencephaly/other severe cranial anomaly. especially ONTD

- Obstructive malformations of GIT, e.g. TOF duodenal stenosis/atresia
- Bone dysplasias.
- Neuromuscular abnormalities.
- Chromosomal abnormality, e.g. trisomy 18.

Salient Features

- Amniotic Fluid Assessment

	Single Pocket	AFI
Oligohydramnios	< 2 cm	< 7
Reduced	2-3 cm	7-10
Normal	3-8 cm	10-17
More than average	> 8-12 cm	17-25
Polyhydramnios	>12 cm	>25

- *Fetal demise:*
  - Fetal wastage after the time significant liquor production is seen leads to slow resorption of liquor.
  - Urine production status at 9 weeks and renal function starts at 11 weeks. At 12 weeks urine accumulates at the rate of 5 cc per day.

- *Signs of IUD are:*
  1. Spalding's sign
     - Overriding of skull bones.
  2. Gas in vessels.
  3. Some times associated hydrops.
  4. Extended limbs/lost tone.
  5. Absent cardiac activity.
  6. Gas in abdomen.

- *IUGR:*
  - Weight of neonate below 10 percentile of the expected fetal weight for that age.
  - Usually detected after 32-34 weeks, i.e. the age of maximum fetal growth.
  - May be due to uteroplacental insufficiency that leads to asymmetric IUGR
  - Asymmetric IUGR is early onset and leads to concordant reduction of all parameters.
  - Criteria for IUGR:

	Sensitivity	Specificity
Advance placental grade	62%	64%
FL/AC (increased)	34-49%	78-83%
TIUV (decreased)	57-80%	72-76%
Small BPD	24-88%	62-94%
Slow increase in BPD	75%	84%
Low EFW	89%	88%
AFV decreased	24%	98%
HC/AC	82%	94%
Biophysical profile	< 6 = Equivocal	
	< 4 = Fetal compromise	

  - Doppler indices
  - Uterine artery—S/D >2.3, difference of the two sides >1, RI > .6
  - MCA –RI < .7
  - Umbilical artery –RI – > .7
- *Post Dated Pregnancy/Large for dates:*
  - When weight is > 90th percentile for the expected fetal weight.
  - Also when weight >4000 gm.
  - Sonographic criteria.

LGA	*Sensitivity*	*Specificity*
• AD/BPD (increase)	46%	79%
• FL/AC (decrease)	24-75%	44-93%
• AFV increase	12-17%	92-98%
• Pondrel index increased	13-15%	85-98%
• High EFW increase	20-74%	93-96%
• Growth score inc.	14%	91%
Macrosomia		
• FL increase	24%	96%
• AC increased	53%	94%
• High EFW	11-65%	89-96%
• BPD increased	29%	98%

- *Renal/bladder abnormality:* Any cause of reduction of urine formation as in renal (B/L) agensis, ARPCKD or of obstruction to outlet of urine as in Prune-Belly syndrome, urethral atresia/stenosis, posterior urethral valve can lead to oligohydramnios. Look for signs of megacystis, i.e. UB > 8 mm, hydronephrosis, i.e. pelvis > 6 mm, abnormal renal parenchyma, dilated ureter and urethra.
- Polyhydramnios occurs when either increased production or decreased fetal galloping of liquor is seen.
- *Cardiovascular decompensation:*

Bradycardia	–	< 100 bpm of >10 sec.
Tachycardia	–	> 180 bpm.
PSVT	–	180-300 bpm with conduction rate 1:1.
Flutter	–	300-400 bpm with conduction rate 2:1/4:1
Fibrillation	–	400 bpm

- *Diaphragmatic hernia:*
  Cystic areas in thorax with small abdomen. Absent fundic bubble, G.B with portal vein pointing up.
- Double bubble and triple bubble sign of duodenal and jejunal ateresia should be looked for.
- Skeletal dysplasia, chromosomal abnormalities detection have been described elsewhere.

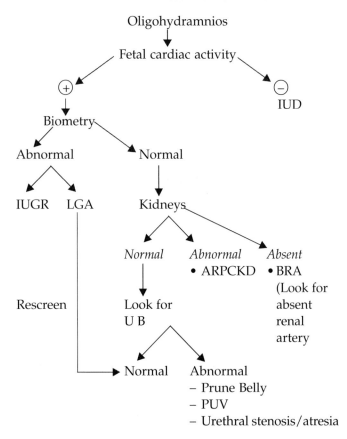

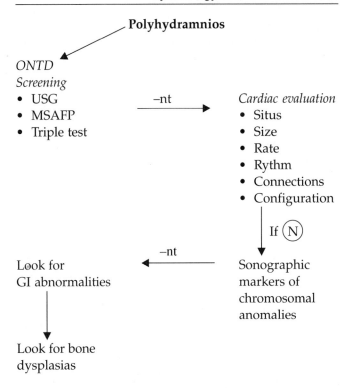

Polyhydramnios

ONTD
Screening
- USG
- MSAFP
- Triple test

−nt →

Cardiac evaluation
- Situs
- Size
- Rate
- Rythm
- Connections
- Configuration

If

Look for
GI abnormalities

←−nt

Sonographic
markers of
chromosomal
anomalies

Look for bone
dysplasias

20.14 INTRA-ABDOMINAL FETAL CALCIFICATION

Causes

A. *Peritoneal:*
   - Meconuim peritonitis.
   - Plastic peritonitis with hydrometrocolpos.
B. *Tumors:*
   - Hemangioma.
   - Hemangioendothelioma.

- Hepatoblastoma.
- Metastatic neuroblastoma.
- Teratoma.

C. *Infections:*
- *Toxoplasma.*
- Cytomegalovirus.

Salient Features

- *Meconuim Peritonitis:*
  - Occurs due to meconuim exiting from the bowel lumen, due to perforation, causing sterile chemical peritonitis.
  - Perforation occurs due to volvulus, jejunal/ileal atresia, meconium ileus.
  - Immediately ascites occurs following which linear streaky or spotty calcification occurs.
  - Pseudocyst formation may also occur.
  - Calcified meconium balls in/out the lumen may also be seen.
- Infections like *Toxoplasma* and CMV lead to calcifications in liver, spleen and also intracranial calcification.
- Hemangiomas may occur at multiple sites in fetal body and may be associated with calcification.
- Hemangioendothelioma and hepatoblastomas
  — Common fetal hepatic tumors which shows areas of specky linear calcification associated with vascular spaces showing high velocity Doppler shifts.
- Hepatoblastoma is the most common hepatic tumor (Primary) in young and nearly all present before the

age of five. Associated with hemihypertropry, 11p13 chromosome and Beckwith-Weidmann's syndrome. Serum AFP levels are almost always elevated. Shows lumpy calcification.

- *Neuroblastoma* is the most common neonatal tumor usually occuring in the adrenal Gland. It is an echogenic mass, heterogenous in appearance.It commonly metastasizes to placenta, liver and subcutaneous tissues with the metastasis appearing Echogenic calcified. Hydrops may commonly occure.

- *Teratomas* and *dermoids* are common fetal tumors occurring in retroperitoneal and gonadal locations most commonly. These show solid and cystic areas with areas of calcification.

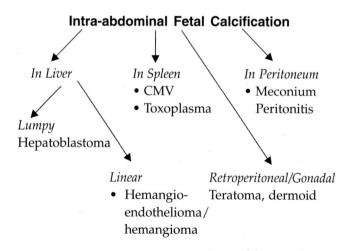

Intra-abdominal Fetal Calcification

In Liver

Lumpy
Hepatoblastoma

In Spleen
- CMV
- Toxoplasma

In Peritoneum
- Meconium
  Peritonitis

Linear
- Hemangio-
  endothelioma/
  hemangioma

Retroperitoneal/Gonadal
Teratoma, dermoid

20.15 D/D OF FETAL THORACIC ABNORMALITIES

Causes

1. Pleural effusion.
2. Congenital diaphragmatic hernias.
3. Pulmonary hypoplasia.
4. Pulmonary sequestration.
5. Pulmonary cystic adenomatoid malformation.
6. Congenital bronchogenic cyst.
7. Bronchial/laryngeal atresia.
8. Thymic enlargment.
9. Cystic hygroma.
10. Teratoma.
11. Enteric cysts.
12. Neuroblastoma.

Salient Features

- Pleural effusion:
    - May be isolated or occur as a result of generalized fetal hydrops.
    - Fluid collects as a crescentic rim around lungs forming a 'Bat-wing-appearance'of lungs floating in fluid.
    - *U/L*—C.A.M, diaphragmatic hernia, sequestration, pulmonary hypoplasia.
    - *B/L*—infections, CHF, Turner's, Downs, Pulmonary lymphangiectasis.
    - Long lasting larger effusions may lead to pulmonary hypoplasia.
    - May be treated by thoracocentesis.

- **Diaphragmatic Hernias:**
  A. *Bochdalak Hernia*
     - Posterolateral in location.
     - Left>>right.
     - Small intestine (88%), stomach (60%), colon (56%), liner (51%),spleen (45%).
     - Detected by sonography at 17 weeks.
     - Mediastinal deviation seen by change in position and axis of heart.
     - Hollow viscera may be seen with AC < 5th percentile and polyhydramnios.
     - Absence of GB in abdomen.
     - Umbilical vein displaced up.
  B. *Morgagni Hernia*
     - Anteriorly behind the sternum.
     - Right>>> left.
     - Omentum, colon, liver, stomach, Small bowel.
     - May be covered by peritoneum and pleura or only pleura or none at all. If pericardium is also absent it lies in direct contact to heart.
  C. *Eventration of Diaphragm*
     - Due to absent muscle fibers in the diaphragm.
     - U/L—asymptomatic.
     - B/L—may cause pulmonary hypoplasia.
     - B/L associated with trisomy 13 and 18, CMV infection, rubella infection and arthrogryposis multiplex congenita.
- **Pulmonary Hypoplasia:**
  - *U/L*—rare, may be simulated by discordant rate of growth of both lungs. Due to thoracic masses.
  - *B/L*—Commoner, due to restricted chest cage as in thanatophoric dwarfism, Jeune's asphyxiating dystrophy, achondrogenesis and all causes of early onset severe oligohydrammios.

$$\frac{\text{Chest area–heart area}}{\text{Chest area}} \times 100$$

is an accurate (85% sensitive and specific) in diagnosis, as correlated to age.

- **Cystic Adenomatoid Malformation**
  - Are hamartomas in lung divided by Adzich in macroscopic (cysts > 5 mm) and microscopic (< 5 mm) types
  - Macroscopic type has better prognosis and is less commonly associated with hydrops.
  - Size of the mass may decrease over the times.
  - Has to be d/d from diaphragmatic hernia, bronchial cyst, cystic dilatation of esophagus, pericardial teratoma.
- **Pulmonary Sequestration**
  - Is a segment or part of lung not communicating at the usually bronchovascular tree.
  - Appears as solid echogenic masses inside (Intralobar sequestration) of the lung. Usually in basal parts.
  - Extralobar may occur inside the diaphragm, pericardium, hila, mediastinum.
  - in 50% malformations of sternum and diaphragm are seen but no major anomaly is seen.
  - D/D to diaphragmatic hernia, CAM and lobar emphysema.
  - A supplying vessel from aorta is the most confirmatory sign.
- Up to 27 weeks the thymus enlarges and appears as echogenic mass (from 14 weeks), after 27 weeks it becomes hypoechoic

- *Cystic hygroma (lymphangiomas)* are cystic (Predominantly) and solid dumb-bell masses extending in the mediastinum
- *Teratomas* usually arise from pericardium and are surrounded by pericardial fluid (diagnostic point). Appearance is the same as in adults
- *Neuroblastomas* are echogenic masses with echolucent centers lying in paravertebral area
- Enteric cyst lined by GI mucosa are also seen in postesior mediastinum.

D/D of Fetal Thoracic Abnormalities

Predominantly Cystic
- Bronchogenic cyst → Solitary
- Dialated esophagus
- Dialated bronchus
- CDH → peristalsis.
- Enteric cyst → posterior
- Meningocele → posterior
- Pericardial cyst

Predeminantly Solid
- CDH → Significant Mediastinal shift
- Sequestration → Vessel from aorta
- CAM (microcystic)
- Teratoma
- Hamartoma
- Ectopic kidney
- Eventration
- Intrathoracic spleen

Solid and Cystic
- CDH → Peristalsis
- CAM → Macrocystic
- Teratoma
- Cystic hygroma
- Eventration
- Neuroblastoma

20.16 UNSUCCESSFUL FIRST TRIMESTER PREGNANCY

Abortion (Miscarriage) — termination of fetus before viability

Type of Embryonic/Fetal loss

1. Complete abortion

USG appearance

Bulky uterus
- Heterogenous vascular myometrium
- Thick heterogenous endometrium
- No products of conception seen

2. Incomplete abortion
- First three features are same as above
- Minimal products of conception especial placenta is retained.

3. Septic
- Apart from above features some foreign body or signs of infection might be noted

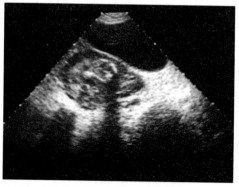

Fig. 20.16.1: Retained products of conception seen in the uterus in a case of incomplete abortion

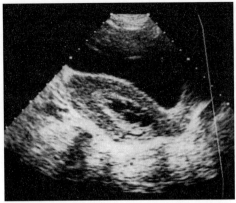

Fig. 20.16.2: Missed abortion—an irregular gestational ring with echoes inside it in normal sized uterus

4. Inevitable/impending/imminent
   - Cervix dialated
   - Membranes protruding
   - Severe pain with uterine contractions
   - Low placed GS, abnormal in shape
5. Missed
   - Whole of products of conception are retained inside for >2 months
   - Fetus is distorted
   - Normal components of conceptus may or may not be identifiable
   - Basically a hetroechoic mass is seen in a bulky uterus but vascularity is reduced.
6. Threatened abortion
   - A normal fetal pole with near normal conceptus noted with the os closed.
   - Basically diagnosed clinically.

Features of Abnormal Gestation Sac

1. Abnormal/irregular shape.
2. Low position
3. Abnormal sac size—most valuable.
   [according to clinicaly judged age].
4. Thin, weakly echogenic, incomplete trophoblastic reaction [< 2 mm].
5. Growth rate is reduced/absent growth on follow up scans.

Abnormal Yolk Sac Features that Suggest Demise

1. Threshold mean sac diameter—must see yolk sac.
   EVS = 8 mm
   TVS = 20 mm
2. Yolk sac size >5.6 mm (5 to 10 week maternal = abnormal outcome age).
3. Calcification in yolk sac.

20.17 FIRST TRIMESTER BLEEDING

1. *With intrauterine conceptus identified*:
   a. Blighted ovum
   b. Vanishing twin syndrome
   c. Implantation bleeding
   d. Threatened abortion
   e. Gestational trophoblastic disease
   f. Ectopic pregnancy with a pseudogestation sac.
2. With empty uterus + beta hCG > 1800 miu/ml:
   a. Recent spontaneous abortion
   b. Ectopic pregnancy

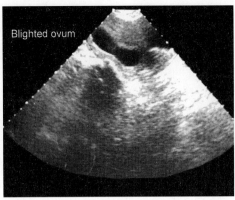

Fig. 20.17.1: Anembryonic gestational sac—no yolk sac is seen in the gestational sac

3. With empty uterus + beta hCG < 1800 miu/ml:
   a. Early intrauterine pregnancy
   b. Ectopic pregnancy.

Blighted Ovum

- Also known as anembryonic pregnancy/embryonic resorption
- Inner cell mass fails to grow further but the sac grows due to persistant trophoblastic function, though suboptimal.
- On USG:
  — Large gestational sac without an embryo
  — Mean sac diameter >16 mm,
     > 25 mm without anembryo
  — Poor sac growth rate
  — Poor perisac trophoblastic reaction
  — Other features of an abnormal sac.

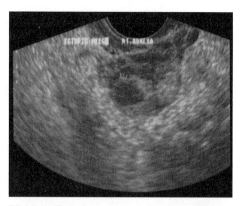

Fig. 20.17.2: Ectopic pregnancy—gray scale image showing a complex right adnexal mass

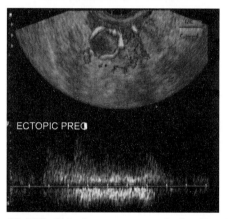

Fig. 20.17.3: Ectopic pregnancy—duplex Doppler demonstrates trophoblastic flow pattern

Ectopic Pregnancy

- Specific features:
  — Live embryo in adnexa

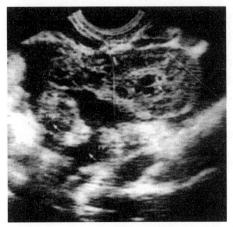

Fig. 20.17.4: Gray scale image showing small ectopic gestation

- Non-specific features (need correlation to beta—hCG)
  - Empty uterus with amenorrhea associated with recent spotting
  - Pseudogestation sac of ectopic pregnancy [created by decidual reaction and associated bleeding], no associated placenta seen.
  - Particulate ascites
  - Adnexal mass—heteroechoic.
  - Ectopic tubal ring—concentric echogenic rim with increased vascularity circumferentially and central hypoechoic area.
  - Adnexal tenderness
  - Interstitial line sign—thin echogenic line from endometrial canal to the ectopic sac.

- Non-supportive features:
  - Live intrauterine pregnancy (as occurrence of heterotopic pregnancy is very rare)
  - Intradecidual sign and double decidual sign of early intrauterine pregnancy.
  - Peritrophoblastic flow.

Gestational Trophoblastic Disease

A. Molar Pregnancy:
   1. Complete mole
   2. Partial mole
B. Persistant Trophoblastic Neoplasia: (PIN)
   1. Invasive mole
   2. Choriocarcinoma
   3. Placental site trophoblastic tumor (PSTT)

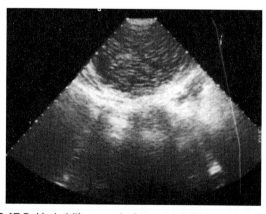

Fig. 20.17.5: Hydatidiform mole (complete). The entire uterus is filled with a heterogeneous mass with multiple anechoic cystic areas in a female with five-month amenorrhea

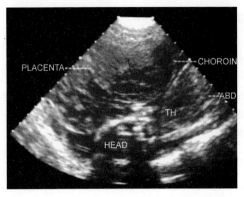

Fig. 20.17.6: Hydatidiform mole (partial)—multiple anechoic spaces in the region of placenta. Fetal parts are seen adjacent to it

On USG

- Echogenic soft tissue interspersed with multiple anechoic areas giving an over all appearance of a spongy mass
  —Snow Storm Appearance
- Perilesional and intralesional vascularity increases in cases of invasive mole, choriocarcinoma, PSTT or any other complication -[RI <.5; PSV >50 cm/s]
- In partial mole, incompletely formed fetal porta may be seen
- In PTN invasion of mass into myometrium is seen.

20.18 FETAL HYDROPS

- Is the abnormal accumulation of fluid in atleast two body cavities
- It represents the terminal stage of a long list of conditions, majority of which are fetal in origin. It signifies fetal decompensation.

Sonographic Features

1. Ascites [> 2 mm] and hydrocele.
2. Pleural effusion.
3. Pericardial effusion (best over cardiac apex].
4. Subcutaneous edema [> 5 mm: Best over scalp].
5. Arterial/venous doppler abnormality.
6. Altered fetal wellbeing.
7. Placental edema [>4-5 cm in third trimester].

Hydrops	
Immune	Non-Immune
• ABO incompatibility • Rh incompatibility • Any other blood group antigen involvement.	• In West, most commonly due to infective, cardiovascular and chromosomal causes in East, thalassemia is most common.

1. Immune Hydrops:
2. On USG-
- Hyperdynamic fetal circulation.
- Enlarged liver and spleen.
- Altered fetal blood parameters:
    — Increasing antibody titer.
    — Amniotic fluid spectrophotometry
    — Fetal blood sampling.
2. Non-immune Hydrops:
A. Fetal causes
    —Cardiovascular:

a. Malformations—cardiac tumors, myocarditis, cardiomyopathy, Ebstein anomaly, endomyocardial fibroelastosis, A-V canal.
b. Arrhythmias—SVT, PAT, WPWS, complete heart block.
c. High output failure—Placental tumors, sacrococcygeal teratoma, vein of Galen aneurysm.

Neck/Thorax Abnormality

- Cystic hygroma
- Thoracic tumor
- Pulmonary sequestration
- Diaphragmatic hernia
- Congenital cystic adenomatoid malformation.

Gastrointestinal Abnormality

- Hepatic—cirrhosis; hepatitis; tumor
- Bowel—atresia; volvulus; meconium peritonitis.

Urinary Tract Abnormality

- Congenital nephrotic syndrome, Prune-Belly syndrome, polycystic kidney disease, upper/lower urinary tract obstruction.

Chromosomal Abnormalities

- 45x, Triploidy, Trisomy 21, 18, 13.

Anemia

Alpha thalassemia (homozygous), HPV B19 infection, G6PD deficiency, fetomaternal hemorrhage, twin-twin transfusion (donor).

Infections

- CMV, HPV, *Toxoplasma*, syphilis, rubella.

Genetic Disorders

- Metabolic—Gaucher's, MPS
- Hypokinesias—AMC, Neu-Laxova, Pena-Shokeir syndrome, mytonic dystrophy.
- Skeletal—achondroplasia, achondrogenesis, asphyxiating thoracic dystrophy, osteogenesis, thanatophoric dysplasia
  —Idiopathic (15-20%)

B. Maternal causes
- Severe anemia
- Severe hypoproteinemia
- Severe diabetes

C. Placental
- Chorioangioma
- Venous thrombosis
- Cord torsion, knot, tumor
  —USG features of above conditions are considered in detailed in relevant topics, in following chapters.

20.19 TWIN PREGNANCY/MULTIFETAL PREGNANCY

Aims of sonography in a clinicaly suspected case of multifetal pregnancy are:

1. To confirm the diagnosis.
2. To determine the chorionicity and amnionicity.
3. To determine the concordance/discordance in growth of fetuses.
4. To determine the complications, if any.
5. To follow up any such case till culminating in a successful outcome.

Sonographic Determination of Chorionicity and Amnionicity:

Step1:   Screen the placenta
- Single placenta = Monochorionic or fused placenta
- > 1 placenta = Dichorionic
- Diamniotic (DCDA)

Step 2:   Screen for a membrane separating the fetuses
- Membrane absent = Monochorionic
- Monoamniotic (MCMA)
- Membrane present = DCDA or MCDA

Step 3:   Determine the fetal sex
- Similar sex = Zygosity cannot be inferred, either MC or DC

Different sex = Dizygotic ∴ Dichorionic

Step 4:   Assess the presence of chorionic/twin peak sign

Present = DCDA

Absent = Equivocal

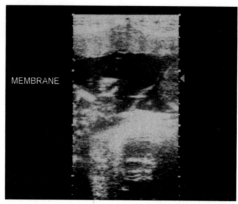

Fig. 20.19.1: A thin echogenic membrane is seen separating the two amniotic sacs in a case of twin pregnancy

Step 5: Thickness of membrane in between
thin = MCDA
thick = DCDA before 22 weeks more reliable
Step 6: Follow the cords from origin and at termination
if reaching a common tangle = MCMA.
Complications of Twin and Multifetal Pregnancy.
A. First trimester pregnancy loss
B. Monochorionic twin syndromes
   a. Twin transfusion syndrome
   b. Twin embolization syndrome
   c. Acardiac parabiotic twin
C. Problems specific to MCMA twins
   a. Conjoined twins
   b. Morbidity/mortality in nonconjoined twins, e.g. cord knotting, cord entanglement
   c. Growth disparity amongs fetuses
   d. Congenital anamolies in fetuses, e.g. CHD, VACTREL, CTEV, torticollis.

Sonographic Features

Twin Transfusion Syndrome (TTS)

- Arterio-venous or arterio-arterial anastomosis in a single placental cotyledon loading to shunting of blood from 'donor' to 'recipient' twin
- Larger twin (Recipient) is normal/Macrosomic while donor is symmetrically growth retarted
- Recipient sac shows polyhydramnios while donor sac shows oligohydramnios
- Donor may even become a 'stuck twin'.
- S/D ratio difference of two sides umbilical artery is > 0.4

Discordant Growth

1. 20-25 percent intrapair birth weight discrepancy.
2. Difference in AC of two of > 18-20 mm.
3. Fetal weight disparity of > 15 percent.
4. Second trimester BPD disparity >5 mm.
5. Umbilical artery S/D disparity > 4.

Twin Embolization Syndrome (TES)

- Demise of co-twin leads to cerebral, hepatic and renal damage of the partner
- Due to exsanguination of live twin, due to embolization from dead twin of debris, clot or thromboplastin rich blood.
- On USG:
   1. Ventriculomegaly.
   2. Porencephaly.

3. Brain atrophy.
4. Microcephaly.
5. Splenic/hepatic infarct.
6. Gut atresias.
7. Facial abnormality.
8. Terminal limb abnormality.
9. Renal cortical necrosis.

Acardiac Parabiotic Twins

- An arterio-arterial or veno-venous placental anastomosis leads to flow reversal in umbilical artery causing poorly oxygenated blood to reach the upper part of body of acardiac twin.
- On USG:
  1. Anencephaly.
  2. Small rudimentary head with holoprosencephaly.
  3. Absent/hypoplastic upper tarso/limbs.
  4. Absent or anomalous two chambered heart.
  5. Cystic hygroma.
  6. Severe oligohydramnios.

Conjoined Twin

On USG:
  1. Continuous, fixed, abnormal/Unusual complimentary position of two twins.
  2. Simultaneous movements.
  3. Common/communicating organs.
  4. Hyperextended head and neck.
Genitourinary System

20.20 D/D OF ECHOGENIC FETAL KIDNEYS

	Conditions	Renal size	Hydro-nephrosis	Liquor	Cyst	Cyst in parents	Family history	Associated features
1.	Infantile polycystic kidney	Large	No	Reduced	No	No	Yes in sibling	Hepatic fibrosis in later life
2.	Adult polycystic	Large	No	Normal	±	Yes, >20 yrs age	Yes in parents liver, spleen	Occasionally cysts in parents
3.	Obstructive cystic dysplasia	Small	Yes	Depends on degree of renal obstruction	Often	No	No	Hydronephrosis usually urethral obstruction
4.	Finnish type nephrotic syndrome	Large	No	Normal	No	No	Yes in sibling	Raised serum AFP
5.	Beckwith-Weidmann syndrome	Large	No	Normal or increased	No	No	±	Macrosomia, Macroglosia, Hepatospleno-megaly, omphalocele

contd...

Contd...

	Condition	Renal size	Hydro-nephrosis	Liquor	Cyst	Cyst in parents	Family history	Associated features
6.	Meckel-Gruber syndrome	Large	No	Reduced	±	No	Yes in sibbling	Polydactyly, enecephalocele
7.	Trisomy	Large	No	Normal	±	No	No	Microcephaly, hydrocephalus, Intracranial calcification, hydrops hepato-splenomegaly
8.	Cytomegalo virus infection	Large	No	Normal	No	No	No	Facial clefting, holoprosence-phaly, poly-dactyly, cardiac defects
9.	Renal vein thrombosis	Large Usually U/L	No	Normal	No	No	No diabetes, maternal pyelonephritis.	Maternal

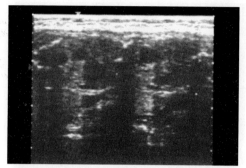

Fig. 20.20.1: Intrauterine hydronephorosis

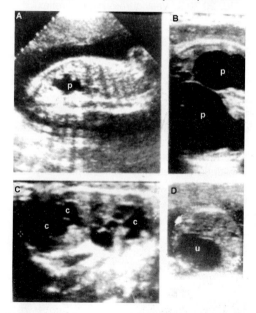

Fig. 20.20.2: PUJ (pelviureteric junction) obstruction: obstruction with variable degree of obstruction P—pelvis, C—calyces, P-U—perinephric urinoma with rupture of calyceal system, seen as unilocular paraspinous cystic mass

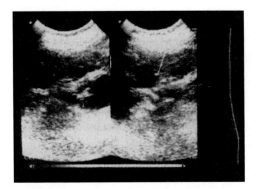

Fig. 20.20.3: Vesicoureteric (VU) reflex

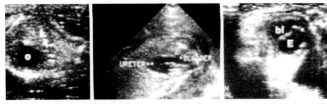

Fig. 20.20.4: Ectopic ureterocoele: Ectopic ureterocoele with ureterectasia to obstructed upper pole resembles a solitary cyst. It's thickened displaced lower lobe parenchyma

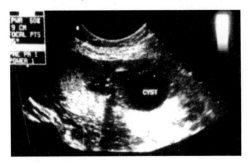

Fig. 20.20.5: Bladder outlet obstruction

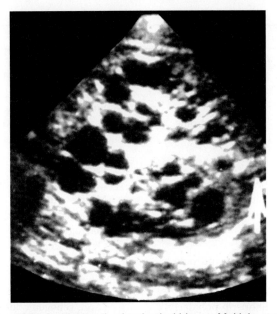

Fig. 20.20.6: Multicystic dysplastic kidney—Multiple cysts seen with no communication

20.21 D/D SYNDROMES ASSOCIATED WITH RENAL MALFORMATIONS

Name and Chief Renal Finding	USG Findings
A. Renal Agenesis:	
a. Fraser syndrome	-Cryptophthalmos -Syndactyly of hand/feet -Large hyperechogenic lungs

Contd...

Table contd...

Name and Chief Renal Finding	USG Findings
B. Cystic Renal Disease:	
a. Meckel Gruber's syndrome	-Large echogenic kidney -Polydactyly. -Encephalocele
b. Patau's syndrome (Trisomy 13)	-Large echogenic kidneys -Polydactyly -Holoprosencephaly -Facial clefting
c. Beckwith Weidmann syndrome	-Large echogenic kidneys -Macrosomia -Hepatosplenomegaly -Macroglossia -Omphalocele
d. Jeune's syndrome	-Echogenic kidney -Small thorax -Dwarfism/I.U.G.R.
e. Short rib polydactyly syndrome (Majewski type)	-Large echogenic kidney -Polydactyly -Small Thorax -Dwarfism/I.U.G.R.
f. Lawrence-Moon-Biedl syndrome (Bardet-Retinal dystrophy	-Renal cyst -Polydactyly -Mental deficiency -Hypogonadism
g. Zellwegger syndrome	-Cystic kidney -Hypotonicity -Limb contractures -Congenital cataract -Heterotopias -Hypoplastic corpus callosum

20.22 D/D OF FETAL HYDRONEPHROSIS

Causes

Unilateral	*Bilateral*
• Pelviureteric junction obstruction	• Pelviureteric junction obstruction
• Vescicoureteric junction obstruction	• Vescicoureteric reflux
• Duplex kidney with ureterocele obstruction	• Vescicoureteric junction
• Normal kidney with ureterocele	• Megacystic megaureter syndrome
• Megaureter	• Posterior urethral valve
	• Urethral atresia
	• Obstructing ureterocele
	• Megacystis microcolon syndrome
	• Congenital megalourethra
	• Persistent cloaca
	• Hydrometrocolpos

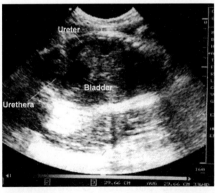

Fig. 20.22.1: Posturethral valve—a longitudinal scan showing dilated posterior urethra, urinary bladder, ureter and left kidney

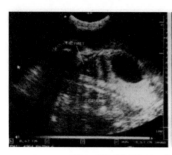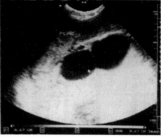

Figs 20.22.2A and B: PUJ obstruction

Dilatation at a median of 19 weeks (in mm) to label hydronephrosis and grading:
- < 4 mm—Normal
- 5-9 mm—Mild
- 10-15—Moderate
- >15—Severe

Pelviureteric Junction Obstruction
- Most common cause
- Males > Females
- 90 percent unilateral

On USG
- Dilated PCS: Normal ureter, bladder
- Renal parenchymal thinning
- Liquor volume normal/increased
- Perinephric urinoma
- Cystic renal dysplasia

Vescicoureteric Junction Obstruction
- Also known as nonrefluxing megaureter

- Male > Female
- 10 percent cases of fetal hydronephrosis.

On USG

- Dilated ureter and PCS
- Bladder and liquor are normal
- No associated bladder outlet obstruction.

Vescicoureteric Reflux

- Female > Male
- Associated with UTI Postanataly
- Prenatal diagnosis more common in boys.

On USG

- Bilateral hydroureteronephrosis with normal liquor volume

Ureterocele/Ectopic Ureter

- Are cystic dilatation of intravescicle segment of ureter

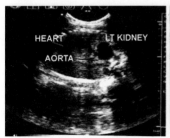 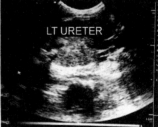

Fig. 20.22.3: Vesicoureteric reflux showing dilated pelvis and dilated ureter

- Associated commonly with duplex collecting system especially in girls. It usually collects the upper moiety
- In boys, it usually drains solitary PCS
- Ectopic ureter may be associated
- Insertions of ectopic ureter are inferomedial to normal opening at trigone, bladder neck, urethra, seminal vescicle, vas deferens, ejaculatory duct, vestibule, vagina, uterus.

On USG

- A large kidney is an indirect evidence of duplex PCS
- Hydroureteronephrosis so gross as to distort the definition of PCS and ureter
- Opposite UVJ may be obstructed by ureterocele
- A ureterocele may prolapse and cause bladder outlet obstruction.
  —Other causes leading to lower urinary tract obstruction are discussed in next section.

20.23 FETAL HEAD, NECK AND FACE

Over 150 different abnormalities of head and face have been described in literature. These can be classified according to the pathogenesis, location of anatomical defects and the structures involved.

Stewart's Classification

1. Otocraniofacial syndromes, i.e. predominantly the ear and mandible involved.

   e.g. Treacher Collins syndrome, Goldenhar syndrome.
2. Facial clefting.
3. Mid face syndromes:
   e.g. Frontonasal dysplasia, holoprosencephalic malformation syndromes.
4. Craniosynostosis syndromes.

20.24 D/D OF MICROGNATHIA

1. Idiopathic: Mild form
2. Chromosomal: Trisomy 18, Triploidy diseases
3. Skeletal dysplasias:
   — Camptomelic dysplasia
   — Diastrophic dysplasia
   — Achondrogenesis
   — Short rib polydactyly syndrome
4. Genetic syndrome:
   — Treacher-Collins syndrome
   — Goldenhar syndrome
   — Hemifacial microsomia
   — Pierre-Robin syndrome
   — Pena-Shokeir syndrome
   — Seckel syndrome
   — Digeorge syndrome
   — Hydrolethalus syndrome
   — Robert's syndrome
   — Mohr's syndrome
   — Miller's syndrome

20.25 D/D OF SYNDROMES ASSOCIATED WITH HYPERTELORISM

1. Frontonasal dysplasia.
2. Frontal encephalocele.
3. Craniosynostosis syndromes.
4. Digeorge syndrome.
5. Hydrolethalus syndrome.
6. Coffin-Lowry syndrome.
7. Noonan's syndrome.
8. Larsen syndrome.
   - 3, 4 and 5 of above are described in relevant sections.

Frontonasal Dysplasia (Median Cleft Syndrome)

A type of mid-facial syndrome

On USG:

1. Marked hypertelorism.
2. Broad, frequently clefted nasal tip.
3. Median cleft lip.

Frontal Encephalocele

- East > West
- 10 percent of all encephaloceles
- Better prognosis
- Brain tissue may herniate into the defect
- Associated agenesis of corpus callosum, hydrocephalus and microcephaly may be seen.
- Anophthalmia may be seen

Coffin-Lowry Syndrome

- Associated with severe mental retardation.

On USG

1. Macroglossia.
2. Hypertelorism.
3. Persistently open mouth.
4. Cavum excavatum.
5. Thoracolumbar scoliosis.

Larsen Syndrome

- May be diagnosed at 20 weeks i/u.

On USG

1. Multiple joint dislocation.
2. Talipes.
3. Abnormal broad thumb, short metacarpals.
4. Hemivertebra/butterfly vertebra.
5. Facial clefting.
6. Cardiac defects.
   - A lethal varient leads to neonatal death due to laryngotracheomalacia and pulmonary hypoplasia. Abnormal palmar creases are seen.

20.26 D/D OF SYNDROMES ASSOCIATED WITH FRONTAL BOSSING

Skeletal Dysplasias

- Achondroplasia

- Achondrogenesis
- Thanatophoric dysplasia.

Craniosynostosis Syndromes

- Crouzon syndrome
- Pfeiffer syndrome
- Craniofrontonasal dysplasia.

Other Syndromes

- Russell silver syndrome
- Robinson syndrome
- Hurler's syndrome
  Described in detail in relevent sections.

20.27 D/D OF SYNDROMES WITH CRANIOSYNOSTOSIS AND OTHER CAUSES

1. Apert's syndrome.
2. Carpenter's syndrome.
3. Crouzon's syndrome.
4. Pfeiffer syndrome.
5. Saethre-Chotzen syndrome.
6. Craniofrontonasal dysplasia.
7. Isolated.

General Features

- Premature fusion of sutures with subsequent limitation of all related structures
- Secondary increase in ICT
- All sutures except metopic (18 months to 2 years) fuse after fourth decade of life

• Premature fusion of	Name
• Sagittal suture	Dolichocephaly
• Coronal suture	Brachycephaly
	Acrocephaly
	turnicephaly
• All sutures+ hydrocephalus	Clover leaf skull

See on next page

20.28 D/D OF CLEFT LIP WITH/ WITHOUT CLEFT PALATE

Chromosomal Defect

- Trisomy 18
- Trisomy 13
- Trisomy 21
- Triploidy

Syndromes and Malformation

- Amniotic band syndrome
- Holoprosencephaly
- Ectodermal dysplasia syndrome
- Robert's syndrome
- Miller's syndrome
- Mohr syndrome
- Frontonasal dysplasia

20.29 D/D OF CONDITIONS ASSOCIATED WITH FACIAL CLEFTING

- Facial clefting is the most common congenital anomalies

Table of Syndromes associated with craniosynostosis

Syndrome	Inheritance	Features	Intelligence
1. Aperts	AD	• Hypertelorism, turnicephaly • Prominent eyes • Syndactyly of toes and fingers (thumb rare)	• 50 percent mental retardation
2. Carpenter	AR	• High forehead, flat facial • Mid facial hypoplasia profile • Polydactyly, preaxial-feet, Post axial-hand	• Variable, can be N, IQ = 54-104
3. Crouzon	AD	Proptosis, hypertelorism, Frontal boss, beak nose, Premature closure of coronal Sutures, ± clover leaf skull of coronal	Usually normal
4. Pfeiffer	AD	Craniosynostosis of coronal, Neurological duplicate big toe, compromise is thumb, Soft tissue syndactyly	Broad common Broad
5. Saethrechotzen	AD	Hypertelorism, mid-face hypoplasia, high-flat forehead, small ears, craniosynostosis of coronal and lambdoid	Most normal
6. CFN dysplasia	XLD	• Female > male, frontal bossing, hypertelorism, syndactyly of fingers and toes	Usually normal

- Asians >> Black
- Males >> Females [except black boys]
- U/L >> B/L : Left >> Right
- Cleft lip and cleft palate are distinct entities and should not be considered as always one.
- Four common combinations of facial clefting is noted:
  1. U/L cleft lip
  2. U/L cleft lip and palate
  3. B/L cleft lip and palate
  4. Isolated cleft palate
- It occurs due to failure of fusion of medial nasal swellings with the maxillary swelling.
  Ultrasound classification of facial clefts

  Normal   Type1
  Type 2   Type 3
  Type 4   Type 5

USG Appearance and Technique

- Antenatal diagnosis can be established in early second trimester but best is to scan at 18-20 week
- A vertical transonic median/paramedian area at upper lip in coronal scanning is noted. This extends to palate if cleft palate is associated
- Bilateral clefting is recognized by the presence of a central echodense mass in the region of upper lip known as premaxillary protrusion. This is best seen in sagittal and axial scanning. This represents abnormal alveolar and gingival tissue resulting from uninhibited growth of the premaxilla caused by lack of continuity of bony, gingival and lip structures.

Isolated Cleft Palate

1. Flow of fluid both in mouth and nasopharynx on color doppler during breathing.
2. Flow of fluid across the palate.
3. Polyhydramnios.
4. Small stomach bubble.
5. Defect in posterior palate noted when the pharynx contains fluid.
   - Once diagnosed, always look for associated anomalies especially cardiac.

Amniotic band syndrome (and limb body wall complex).
- Early amnion rupture allows fetus to enter the chorionic cavity ∴ entrapping the fetal parts amongst the fibrous septa that traverse this cavity.

On USG
1. Type 5 (usually) facial clefts.
2. Paramedian encephaloceles.
3. Gastropleuroschiasis.
4. Limb amputation defects.
5. Spinal curvature abnormality.
   - Abdominal wall defect + spinal curvature defect—deagnostic.

Ectrodactyly-Ectodermal Dysplasia-Clefting Syndrome (EEC)

- AD

On USG

1. Lobster claw deformity.
2. Hydronephrosis, VUR.
3. Cleft lip/palate.

Robert's Syndrome

- A.D: lethal in neonates: Premature centromere separation (chromosome puffs) in centromeric staining is diagnostic

On USG

1. Cleft lip with/without cleft palate.
2. Micrognathia.
3. Prominent premaxilla.
4. Preminent eyes.
5. Malformed ears.
6. Limb reduction defects (more severe in upper limb).
7. Congenital heart disease.
8. Cystic dysplasia of kidneys.

Miller Syndrome (Acrofacial Dysostosis with Postaxial Defects)

- AR

On USG

1. Micrognathia.
2. Cleft lip.
3. Prominent eyes.
4. Absent fith digit in all four limbs.
5. Ulnar/radial hypoplasia with incurving forearm.

MOHR Syndrome (Orofacial Digital Syndrome)

- AR
- Can be diagnosed as early as 20 weeks

On USG

1. Median cleft lip.
2. Micrognathia.
3. High/cleft palate.
4. Post-axial polydactyly in hand and feet and pre-axial also in feet.
5. Severely hypoplastic tibia.

20.30 FETAL CENTRAL NERVOUS SYSTEM

- CNS abnormalities are the most common cause of referal for prenatal diagnosis
  Ventriculomegaly and hydrocephalus
- Enlargement of ventricles is refered to as ventriculomegaly while above when associated with increased intracranial tension and/or head enlargement is known as hydrocephalus.

On USG

1. Occipital horn > 10 mm.
2. Distance of medial ventricular wall from medial border of choroid is >3 mm.
3. Total distance between lateral edges of the two anterior horns > 20 mm [at GA < 24 weeks and at BPD < 6.5 mm].
4. Ventricle to hemisphere ratio as correlated to gestational age from namograms [35% at 25 week].
5. Difference of >3 mm in the size of two atria.
6. Convex wall at anterior horns.
7. Asymmetry of choroids.

8. 'Droopy' or 'dangling' choroids.
9. Undulating septum pellucidum.

Acrania, Anencephaly, Exencephaly

- Acrania = Absent cranial vault with a normal brain matter
- Anencephaly = Acrania with absence of cerebral hemispheres and diencephalic structures which are replaced by an amorphus mass of neurovascular tissue known as area cerebrovasculosum orbits and face are normal.
- Exencephaly = The amorphus mass described above is identifiable with the normal brain matter
- Cranioschiasis = Dysraphic abnormality involves the head and entire spine
  — Above abnormalities are associated with spinal, non-CNS abnormalities and polyhydramnios
  — These should not be diagnosed with confidence until 11½ weeks when ossification of frontal bones is visible using TVS. The diagnosis is made with 100 percent confidence only after 14 weeks.
  — D/D-Amniotic band syndrome
    — Large encephaloceles

Encephaloceles including Cephaloceles, Myeloceles, etc

- Are herniations of any part of neural tube through a defect in adjoining part of skull and spine
- Nomenclature depends on the exact site of defect and the part of neural tube protruding.

- Seen as a cystic mass that may or may not contain echogenic internal contents
- Meckel-Gruber's syndrome is a lethal autosomal recessive condition characterized by polydactyly postaxial (in 55% cases)
  — Occipital cephalocele (60 to 85%),
  Polycystic kidneys (100%). Microcephaly may be an associated feature.
- D/D-Cystic hygroma
  — Hemangioma
  — Teratoma
  — Branchial cleft cyst
  — Scalp edema.

Spina Bifida

Sonographic signs include:-
1. Lemon sign—seen mostly < 24 week
   — Bifrontal indentations.
2. Ventriculomegaly.
3. Banana sign—obliterated cisterna magna with a smoothly convex posterior cerebellar margine without the bilobbed configuration.
4. Spinal defect with cystic mass.
5. Slightly smaller fetal head measurement.

Iniencephaly

- Dysraphism involving the back of cranium and contiguous upper spine
- A short neck with star gazing position of child
- Associated anencephaly, Kippel Feil syndrome may be seen.

Abnormal Cisterna Magna

- Normal size (Anteroposterior) is 4-10 mm
- Small in Arnold-Chiari malformation
- Enlarged in: Normal variant
  — Tonsillar/cerebellar hypoplasia
  — Communicating hydrocephalus
  — Arachnoid cyst
    Dandy-Walker cyst
  — Trisomy 18.

Holoprosencephaly

1. Hypotelorism.
2. Midline maxillary cleft.
3. Cyclopia (Single eye with supraorbital proboscis).
4. Ethmocephaly (hypotelorism with proboscis).
5. Cebocephaly (hypotelorism with single nostril).
6. Alobar type:
   — Cup type—anterior cup like cerebral mantle with a dorsal cyst.
   — Pancake type—anterior small plate like cerbrum with a large dorsal cyst
   — Ball type—single featureless
     — Monoventricle surrounded by a mantle of varying width.
7. Semilobar type:
   - Rudimentary occipital horns seen.
8. Lobar type:
   - Absent cavum septum pellucidum
   - Fusion and squaring of frontal horns
   - Rudimentary, fused, abnormal shaped fornices.

- D/D—hydrocephalus
  — hydranencephaly

Dandy Walker Malformation

Diagnosed at >18 weeks
1. Vermian agenesis/hypoplasia.
2. Posterior fossa cyst communicating to fourth ventricle.
3. Elevated tentorium.
4. Ventriculomegaly.
5. Agenesis of corpus collosum.
6. Congenital heart disease.
7. Polydactyly.
8. Genitourinary abnormality.
- D/D -Arachnoid cyst
  — Megacisterna magna.

Hydranencephaly

1. Supraclinoid carotid system not seen.
2. No cortical mantle seen.
3. Large fluid filled cavities seen in head.
4. Head size commonly normal.
   - D/D—severe hydrocephalus
     — Alobar holoprosencephaly
     — Massive congenital subdural hygroma.

Schizencephaly

- On USG, cleft which may be bilateral and symmetrical are noted mainly in parietal and temporal areas
- Such clefts are smooth and lined by gray matter.

Lissencephaly [agyria]

Diagnosed after 28 week
1. Mild ventriculomegaly.
2. Large, open Sylvian fissure.
3. Abnormal corpus callosum.
4. Gyri are absent or broad and flat know as pachy-gyria.

Micro/Macrocephaly

- Head size (BPD) below or above 3 SD of normal for that particular age and sex
- Also altered are:
  1. Head circumference
  2. HC: AC
  3. FL: HC
  4. Frontal lobe size.

Agenesis of Corpus Callosum

1. Disproportionately large occipital horns known as colpocephaly.
2. Lateral displacement of both medial and lateral ventricular wall.
3. Steer horn shapped frontal horns.
4. Interhemispheric cyst/lipoma.
5. Sunray like sulci and gyri radiating to ventricular margine.
6. Third ventricles is high placed and projects between lateral ventricles.

Aqueductal Stenosis

- Large lateral and third ventricles with thinned parenchyma

- Isolated, nonprogressive abnormality.

Space Occupying Lesions

1. Arachnoid cyst.
2. Choroid plexus cyst.
3. Vein of Galen aneurysm.
4. Teratoma.
5. Glioblastoma.
6. Craniopharyngioma.
7. Neuroblastoma.
8. Subependymal hamartomas.

No specific imaging features are noted, the location is the primary diagnostic feature.

Sacrococcygeal Teratoma

1. Mass in rump/buttocks.
2. Solid/solid+cystic.
3. Calcification frequent.
4. Displaced/distorted adjacent structures.
5. Hydronephrosis.
6. Fetal cardiac failure/hydrops.
7. Size < 4.5 cm—advice elective vaginal delivery
   >4.5 cm—advice cesarean.
   —D/D
      — Chordoma
      — Anterior myelomeningocele
      — Neuroenteric cyst
      — Neuroblastoma
      — Bone tumor
      — Lymphoma
      — Rectal duplication

— Lipoma
— Sarcoma.

Caudal Regression Syndrome

- Ranging in severity from absence of sacrum (or only a part of it) to absence of whole lumbar spine
- Hypoplastic leg, oligohydramnios
- More common (25 times) in diabetic mothers
- Associated abnormalities are VACTREL, kyphoscoliosis, pelvic bone deformity, CTEV
- Severest form if sirenomelia:
  1. Absent sacrum.
  2. Fused legs.
  3. Anorectal atresia.
  4. Renal agenesis/dysgenesis.
  5. Cardiac defects:
     This is also known as Mermaid syndrome.

Diastematomyelia

1. Sagittal cleft in spinal cord/conus/filum.
2. Hydromyelia.
3. Spina bifida.
4. Fibrous/bony sagittal septum.

Myelocystocele

1. Dilated central canal.
2. Spina bifida may be absent.
3. Sac present posteriorly consists of skin, meninges and ependyma lined hydromyelia sac.
   The overall appearance is known as the 'Cyst within Cyst'.

20.31 FETAL ABDOMINAL WALL DEFECTS

1. Gastroschisis.
2. Omphalocele.
3. Pentalogy of Cantrell.
4. Limb-body wall complex known as body stalk abnormality.
5. Bladder and cloacal extrophy.

SONOGRAPHIC FEATURES

Gastroschisis

1. Full thickness abdominal wall defect.
2. Paraumbilical location (usually right) of the defect.
3. Small size (2-4 cm).
4. Free floating bowel loops in amniotic fluid.
5. No enveloping membrane.

Omphalocele

1. Central anterior abdominal wall defect containing bowel/solid viscera.
2. Mass encompassed by umbilical cord.
3. Limiting membrane covering the defect.

Pentalogy of Cantrell

1. Midline anterior wall defect usually involving the upper abdomen.
2. Ectopic heart.
3. Pericardial/pleural effusion.
4. Craniofacial abnormality.
5. Ascites.

6. Two-vessel-cord.
7. Omphalocele.

Limb-Body-Wall Complex

1. Large ventral wall defect (usually left sided) of the abdomen and thorax.
2. Craniofacial abnormality.
3. Marked scoliosis and/or spinal dysraphism .
4. Limb defects.
5. Short or absent umbilical cord.
6. Amniotic bands.

Cloacal Extrophy

1. Large infraumbilical anterior wall defect with irregular anterior wall mass.
2. Absent bladder.
3. Malformation of the genitalia.
4. May be neural tube defects.

For table see on next page

Table 20.31.1: Fetal abdominal wall defects

	Gastroschisis	Omphalocele	Limb-body wall complex	Cloacal extrophy
1. Location	Right paraumbilical	Infraumbilical insertion site	Midline, at cord left	Lateral, usually
2. Size of defect	Small (2-4 cm)	Variable (2-10 cm)	Large	Variable
3. Membrane	—	+	+ (contiguous to placenta)	Variable
4. Liver involvement	—	Common	+	+
5. Ascites	—	Common	—	Variable
6. Bowel thickening and dilatation	+	—	—	Variable (unless ruptured)
7. Bowel complications	Common	—	—	—
8. Cardiac	Rare abnormalities	Common (ASD, PDA) (complex)	Common	10-15 percent
9. Chromosomal abnormalities	—	Common	—	Variable
10. MS-AFP	+	+/−		Always
11. Other abnormalities	Rare	Common	Always (scoliosis, cranial defect, limb defects)	Genitourinary, spinal

20.32 NUCHAL FOLD AND TRANSLUSCENCY

	Nuchal Fold Thickness	*Transluscency*
1. Measurement section	Axial; thalmii, occipital bone and cerebellum seen	Sagittal; Midsagittal section of head
2. From-to	Outer edge of bone to outer interface	Outer edge of bone to subcutaneous surface of skin
3. Normal measurement with GA	14-18 week >5 mm-abnormal 4-5 mm-borderline <4 mm-Normal 18-22 week > 6 mm-abnormal 5-6 mm-borderline <5 mm-Normal	10-14 week > 3 mm is abnormal At 10-12 week 1.5 mm = 50th percentile 2.5 mm = 95th percentile At 12-14 week 2 mm = 50th percentile 3 mm = 95th percentile
4. Indicate	• Trisomy 21	• Cardiac abnormality • Chromosomal abnormality (18,13,21) • Cystic hygroma

20.33 PRENATAL SONOGRAPHIC DIAGNOSIS OF CARDIAC ANOMALIES

Common indications for fetal echocardiogram:

1. Abnormal four chambered view on screening USG.
2. Fetal hydrops.
3. Polyhydramnios.
4. Fetal arrhythmias.
5. Chromosomal abnormalities.
6. Extracardiac abnormalities.

7. Family history of CHD/syndromes associated with CHD.
8. Maternal diseases as diabetes, phenylketonuria, collagen vascular diseases.
9. Teratogen exposure (Rubella, alcohol, drugs).
10. Monitoring responce to intrauterine therapy.
11. Monitoring fetus at risk for decompunsation in cases of hydrops, persistant tachyarrhythmias.

Best Timing for Echocardiography

- Is 18-22 weeks, as before 18 weeks heart is very small while after 22 weeks bony shadow, less liquor, awkward fetal position limit the examination
- With vaginal probe the procedure may be done as early as 12-13 weeks.

STRUCTURAL DEFECTS

Atrial Septal Defects

- Arises after 4-6 weeks
- On USG:
  1. Difficult to distinguish small pathologic ASD from PFO.
  2. A PFO is about 1 mm less than the aortic root diameter while ASD is larger than this.
  3. The primum ASD is low placed in atrial septum near AV valve.

Ventricular Septal Defect

- Highest recurrance rate
- Most teratogen associated defect

On USG

1. An area of discontinuity in interventricular septum
2. On color Doppler, bidirectional interventricular shunting with a systolic right to left and late diastolic left to right shunt.
3. Unidirectional shunting indicates additional abnormalities.

Atrioventricular Septal Defects

- Occurs due to malformation in atrioventricular cushion

On USG

1. Defect in atrial and/or ventricular septum.
2. Single abnormal A-V valve seen.
3. Demonstration of bridging leaflet is a confirmatory evidence of incomplete type AVSD.
4. Color Doppler shows a defect across endocardial cushion and abnormal A-V valve with valvular insufficiency.
5. A left ventricle to right atrial jet may be seen.
6. Holosystolic insufficiency on color Doppler is a late but ominous abnormality.

Ebstein Anomaly

- Inferior displacement of the tricuspid valve, frequently with leathered attachment of leaflets, tricuspid dysplasia and right ventricular dysplasia.
- Most commonly associated to maternal lithium exposure.

On USG

1. Apical displacement of tricuspid valve in right ventricle.
2. Enlarged right atrium containing a part of atrialized right ventricle.
3. Reduction in size of atrialized right ventricle.
4. TR seen on color Doppler.
5. M-mode shows presence of arrhythmias especially supraventricular tachycardias.

Hypoplastic Right/Left Heart Syndromes

• Hypoplasia of ventricle due to inflow reduction (Tricuspid/mitral atresia) or due to outflow reduction [Pulmonary/aortic reduction]

On USG

1. Small respective ventricle with concentric hypertrophy.
2. Hypoplastic/atretic respective inflow and/or outflow channels.
3. On color Doppler, single area of flow at A-V valve level. A decreased flow is seen if only hypoplasia of channels is present.
4. Associated arrhythmias and CHF may be seen

Univentricle Heart

• Due to failure of developement of interventricular septum a single ventricle, having LV morphology, but no outflow tract (type B) or common outflow tract (type A) is seen

On USG

1. Single ventricle with absent interventricular septum
2. Color Doppler is used to confirm or refute the presence of an outflow tract ∴ d/d between type A and B.

Tetralogy of Fallot

- Due to far anterior placement of conus septum thus dividing the conus into smaller anterior right ventricular portion and a large posterior part. Closure of interventricular septum is thus incomplete leading to aortic over-riding.
- Diagnosis can be made on or before 15 weeks using EVS probe

On USG

1. Perimembranous VSD.
2. Dilated aorta.

Persistent Truncus Arteriosus

- A single large vessel arises from base of heart sypplying coronary, systemic and arterial circulations
- VSD is almost always associated
- Truncal valve has two to six cusps and over-rides the ventricular septum
- On USG: around 15 weeks
  1. Above described defects seen.
  2. Color Doppler is very helpful in localizing pulmonary arterial and estimating the presence of insufficiency.

Double Outlet Right Ventricle

- More than 50 percent of both aorta and pulmonary artery arise from right ventricle

On USG

1. Above defects are noted. Three types seen:
   a. Aorta posterior and right to pulmonary artery.
   b. Both parallel with aorta to the right (Taussig-Bing syndrome).
   c. Both parallel with the aorta anterior and to the left.

Transposition of Great Arteries

Two types:
A. Complete or dextrotransposition (D-TGA)
- Atrioventricular concordance with ventriculo-arterial discordance
  — VSD present (30%)
  — VSD absent (70%)
B. Congenitally corrected or levotransposition (L-TGA)
- Atrioventricular discordance with ventriculoarterial discordance
- On USG
  1. Great vessels exit the heart parallel to each other rather than crossing.
  2. Color Doppler characterizes the flow.

Anomalous Pulmonary Venous Return

- Due to failure of obliteration of normal embryological connections between the primitive pulmonary veins and the splanchnic, umbilical, vitelline and umbilical veins such that none or only few pulmonary veins drain into left atrium.

On USG

1. Mild prominence of right ventricle and pulmonary artery
2. On duplex Doppler, a ratio of right to left flow of >2 percent
3. Small left atrium

Coarctation of Aorta

On USG

1. Right to left ventricle diameter ratio more than 2 SD above the normal.
2. Pulmonary artery to ascending aorta diameter ratio above 2 SD than normal.
3. Presence of distal aortic arch hypoplasia.

Cardiosplenic Syndromes

- Are defects of lateralization in which symmetric developement of normally asymmetric organ/organ system occur.

A. *Asplenia (Bilateral Right Sidedness):*
   1. Right atrial isomerism.
   2. Bilateral trilobed lung.
   3. Bilateral right bronchii.
   4. Bilateral right pulmonary arteries.
   5. Ipsilateral location of aorta and IVC.

6. Absence of spleen.
7. Midline horizontal liver.
8. Bilateral superior vena cava.
9. Severe and complex heart abnormalities.
B. *Polysplenia (Bilateral Left Sidedness)*
   1. Interruption of IVC.
   2. Azygous continuation of IVC.
   3. Multiple spleens.
   4. Left atrial isomerism.
   5. Complete A-V block.

Cardiac Tumors

75 percent—Rhabdomyoma
19 percent—Teratoma
12 percent—Fibroma
2 percent—Cardiac hemangioma
2 percent—Mesothelioma of A-V node
Rhabdomyoma
— Single/multiple
— Project in the cavity
— From interventricular septum
— 30-78 percent have tuberus sclerosis

Teratoma

Solid + cystic

Ectopia Cordis

- Due to failure of fusion of the lateral body fold in the thoracic region
- Heart located out of thorax
- May be a part of pentalogy of Cantrell

Arrhythmias (diagnosed on M-Mode)

1. Premature atrial/ventricular
2. Tachycardia:
   - Heart rate >180 bpm
   - Mostly supraventricular
   - 4 types:
     — 180-300 bpm with conduction
     — rate 1:1 = PSVT
     — 300-400 bpm + 2:1/4:1
     — = flutter
   > 400 bpm atrial rate + ventricular rate 120-160 Bpm
     — = Fibriltation
3. Bradycardia:
   prolonged heart rate < 100 bpm for >10 seconds.

Index